MCQs for the Pr

MCQs for the Primary FRCA

B.S.K. Kamath
MB, BS, DA, FRCA *former Consultant, Barnet Hospital Trust*

Sarah Turle
MB, ChB, FRCA, *Specialty Registrar, Central London School of Anaesthesia*

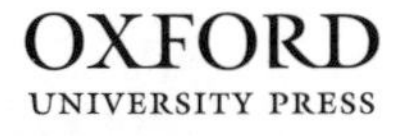
OXFORD
UNIVERSITY PRESS

OXFORD
UNIVERSITY PRESS

Great Clarendon Street, Oxford OX2 6DP

Oxford University Press is a department of the University of Oxford.
It furthers the University's objective of excellence in research, scholarship, and education by publishing worldwide in

Oxford New York

Auckland Cape Town Dar es Salaam Hong Kong Karachi
Kuala Lumpur Madrid Melbourne Mexico City Nairobi
New Delhi Shanghai Taipei Toronto

With offices in

Argentina Austria Brazil Chile Czech Republic France Greece
Guatemala Hungary Italy Japan Poland Portugal Singapore
South Korea Switzerland Thailand Turkey Ukraine Vietnam

Published in the United States
by Oxford University Press Inc., New York

First published 2010

British Library Cataloguing in Publication Data
Data available

Library of Congress Cataloguing in Publication Data
Data available

Typeset by Glyph International, Bangalore, India
Printed in Great Britain
on acid-free paper by
the MPG Books Group, Bodmin and King's Lynn

ISBN 978–0–19–957577–0

9 8 7 6 5 4 3 2

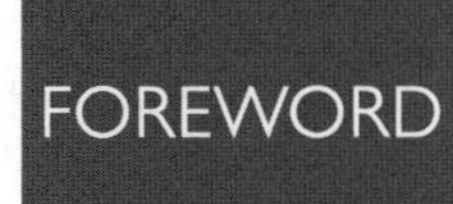

FOREWORD

In 35 years of taking examinations, helping prepare candidates for examinations, and being involved in the conduct of examinations, I have yet to meet one person who likes multiple-choice questions (MCQs). Not one. These interrogative instruments of torture seem to be universally reviled by candidates throughout the world and from all academic disciplines, and yet examiners and those with expertise in the science of examination tell us that they are a reliable and repeatable method of assessing true knowledge. The practice of anaesthesia may well be an art, but it is an art that is based on detailed scientific knowledge drawn from a variety of disciplines. The nascent anaesthetist must therefore have a good working knowledge of what are sometimes the drier aspects of physics, pharmacology, and physiology. Indeed, it is the breadth and depth of this knowledge that sets anaesthetists apart from many other medical specialties. Perhaps sadly, almost all of this technical underpinning to the safe practice of anaesthesia is fiercely factual, and this knowledge is therefore highly amenable to assessment by the dreaded MCQ. Add to this the ease with which a computer armed with a simple optical interface can check the answers and provide the results to the examiner, and you have a malevolent match made in heaven: the Primary FRCA and the MCQ. Many hours of hard work at a computer or reading a textbook is undoubtedly the secret to acquiring the knowledge required to pass this exam, but an equally important support to success is practice. That's practice as in practice, practice, practice. Answering large numbers of MCQs during preparation for the Primary FRCA not only hones one's ability to respond to these little challenges, but it also highlights areas in which one's knowledge may be slightly—or sometimes even completely—lacking before the day of judgement arrives. This book, written by two experienced anaesthetists with a very firm grasp of the subjects involved in the Primary FRCA, not only poses the candidate questions that cover all the relevant areas in physics, pharmacology, and physiology covered by the exam, and provides answers to MCQs posed, but it also offers explanations of the answers that can lead to further reading if the candidate feels that this is necessary. It is an excellent book and an excellent way of preparing for the examination. I would strongly recommend that all Primary FRCA candidates invest in this book and go through it in a logical, methodical and enquiring way.

Having attended Primary FRCA viva and OSCE days on more than one occasion, I can thoroughly support the often proposed but rarely believed view (by candidates at least) that the examiners try very hard to pass candidates. It's true – they really are on your side and will pass you if you let them. However, even without negative marking, the MCQ is a cold and dispassionate assessment tool that cannot make allowances for lack of experience or excess of anxiety. You therefore need to read and to practice to pass the MCQ paper.

And then practice a little more.
Good luck!

Dr William Harrop-Griffiths
Consultant Anaesthetist, St Mary's Hospital, Imperial College Healthcare NHS Trust, London

For my family
BSKK

For all my family, especially Paul
ST

ACKNOWLEDGEMENTS

We would like to thank Christopher Reid and Stephanie Ireland of Oxford University Press for all of their help during the preparation of this book. We are also extremely grateful to Dr William Harrop-Griffiths for giving his time and attention in reviewing the book and also for writing the foreword.

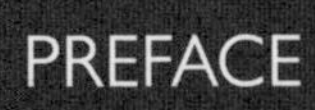

PREFACE

In order to be successful in the multiple-choice question (MCQ) section of the Primary FRCA, candidates have been always required to have an in depth knowledge of the syllabus encompassing pharmacology, physics and clinical measurement, and physiology.

Knowledge has become even more crucial now that there has been a change to the way the MCQ section is marked. Whereas previously the negative marking approach of the examination required a more tactical technique, it is now necessary to attempt every question and score in the region of 75% to pass.

We have designed this MCQ book with the new style of examination in mind. The book is set out as four complete papers with 90 questions in each paper, comprising 30 questions each in pharmacology, physics and clinical measurement, and physiology. This way the user can easily attempt a paper that resembles the real examination under timed conditions. Earlier in the revision, the user may alternatively wish to concentrate on particular areas of the syllabus, and the book is set out to facilitate this.

We have included a full answer for each subsection of each question, so that the candidate can enhance their knowledge, and we have also included diagrams and figures to help illustrate key topics. We feel that certain areas such as respiratory physiology require special attention, as these are recurring themes that are prominent in both the MCQ and the structured oral examination (SOE) sections of the Primary FRCA. We have included questions that may be asked in the light of the development of new drugs, techniques, and equipment. For the user who is keen to develop their knowledge further, there are references at the end of each question, which we hope will make revision easier.

It is easy to feel overwhelmed at the sheer volume of knowledge required in order to pass the examination, but certain points should be borne in mind. There is no secret to success in this examination, but one can be prepared by having a sound knowledge base, and by doing lots and lots of practice. Lastly, it is worth remembering the golden rules of MCQs, which state 'never say never and never say always' and 'always read the question thoroughly'.

Good luck!
BSKK
ST

CONTENTS

chapter 1

PHARMACOLOGY

QUESTIONS

1 Suxamethonium:

- a Is a dicholine ester of succinic acid
- b Has a quaternary ammonium group at each end of the molecular chain
- c Does not cause histamine release
- d Can be hydrolysed in the complete absence of serum cholinesterase
- e Does not cause malignant hyperpyrexia if a trigger agent such as isoflurane is not used

2 Morphine:

- a In a dose of 15 mg provides equal analgesic effect as inhaled 30% nitrous oxide
- b Depresses antidiuretic hormone (ADH) secretion
- c May exacerbate biliary colic
- d Depresses gastric motility
- e Depresses the chemoreceptor trigger zone (CTZ)

3 Ranitidine:

- a Is a H_1 receptor antagonist
- b Reduces gastric acidity as well as the volume of gastric secretions
- c Is given in a dose of 150 mg intravenously
- d Inhibits cytochrome P450
- e Is contraindicated in porphyria

4 Regarding ultra-short-acting barbiturates:

- a They are modified compounds of malonyl urea
- b They are mainly metabolized by the kidney
- c They decrease cerebral oxygen consumption
- d Respiratory alkalosis decreases their duration of action
- e Metabolic alkalosis increases their rate of renal excretion

5 Hydantoin derivatives:

- a Are closely related in structure to barbiturates
- b Have a membrane-stabilizing effect
- c Produce generalized central nervous system (CNS) depression
- d May be used in the treatment of certain cardiac dysrhythmias
- e Include one of the drugs used in the management of malignant hyperpyrexia

6 Diuretic therapy leads to:

a Hypochloraemic acidosis with bendroflumethiazide
b Metabolic alkalosis with carbonic anhydrase inhibitors
c Hyperuricaemia with thiazides
d Hyperglycaemia with bumetanide
e Hypokalaemia with amiloride

7 Cocaine:

a Is an amide
b Was the first local anaesthetic agent to be used
c Can be used as a surface anaesthetic
d May cause raised body temperature
e May cause hypertension

8 Thiopental (thiopentone):

a Has a pH of 8.2
b Is the sulphur analogue of pentobarbitone
c Is greater than 60% bound to plasma proteins after intravenous (IV) administration
d Diffuses rapidly into fatty tissues two minutes after IV administration
e Can produce a demyelination syndrome in susceptible individuals

9 The following are potassium-sparing diuretics:

a Acetazolamide
b Furosemide
c Thiazides
d Spironolactone
e Amiloride

10 Regarding local anaesthetic drugs:

a Absorption is better from the trachea than the pharynx following topical application
b They are inactivated in tissues with a high pH
c Methaemoglobin may be formed following the use of certain drugs
d Heavy bupivacaine contains 6% dextrose to make it heavier than cerebrospinal fluid (CSF)
e The pseudocholinesterase assay is performed using a local anaesthetic drug

11 The following drugs reduce afterload:

a Aminophylline
b Labetalol
c Glyceryl trinitrate
d Isoprenaline
e Noradrenaline (norepinephrine)

12 Following are examples of competitive antagonism:

a Tubocurarine and acetylcholine
b Salicylates and oral hypoglycaemics
c Barbiturates and oral anticoagulants
d Naloxone and opiates
e Chlorpromazine and dopamine

13 Administration of the following may decrease renal blood flow:

a Theophylline
b Ephedrine
c Cyclopropane
d Isoprenaline
e Dobutamine

14 Remifentanil:

a Is an ultra-short-acting opioid
b Is hydrolysed by pseudocholine esterase
c Effects lasts for 15–20 minutes
d Causes muscle rigidity
e Can be used in a patient-controlled analgesia (PCA) regimen in labour

15 Nicotinic actions of acetylcholine include:

a Increased salivation
b Bronchospasm
c Bradycardia
d Control of muscle contraction
e CNS excitation

16 Isoflurane:

a Has boiling point of 60°C
b Has a minimum alveolar concentration (MAC) of 0.75
c Is metabolized into trifluoroacetic acid in the liver
d Has a saturated vapour pressure of 33 kPa at 20°C
e Contains thymol as a preservative in the bottle

17 Therapeutic excess of oral anticoagulants may be reversed with:

a Aprotinin
b Vitamin K
c Human albumin solution (HAS)
d Fresh frozen plasma
e Cryoprecipitate

18 Ganglion blocking drugs produce:

a Hypotension
b Miosis
c Increased tone of intestinal muscles
d Bradycardia
e Increased sweating

19 Drugs used in diagnosis or treatment of myasthenia gravis include:

a Edrophonium
b Pralidoxime
c Amantadine
d Decamethonium
e Aminopyridine

20 Glycopyrrolate:

a Is an anticholinergic agent that can produce significant sedation
b In a 500 μg dose is added to neostigmine and used for the reversal of neuromuscular blocking drugs
c Increases intraocular pressure
d It may be used safely in children as well as adults
e May produce supraventricular arrhythmias

21 Derivatives of opium include:

a Methadone
b Pethidine
c Dextropropoxyphene
d Codeine
e Papaveretum

22 Cyanide poisoning:

a May result from excess infusion of glyceryl trinitrate
b Increases the arterio-venous oxygen gradient
c Decreases the partial pressure of oxygen
d Increases the arterial pH
e Should be treated with methylene blue because methaemoglobin has more affinity for cyanide than normal haemoglobin

23 Drugs producing bronchodilation include:

a Xanthine derivatives
b Muscarine
c Pilocarpine
d 5-hydroxytryptamine
e Diethyl ether

24 Adverse effects of nitrous oxide include:

- a Loss of hearing
- b Bone marrow aplasia
- c Diffusion hypoxia
- d Pulmonary oedema, if contaminated with its higher oxide
- e Cranial nerve palsy

25 Induction is more rapid with an inhalational agent:

- a If it has a low blood/gas partition coefficient
- b If it has a high oil/gas coefficient
- c If carbon dioxide is administered during the early phase of induction
- d If controlled ventilation is employed
- e In old age

26 Alkaline diuresis promotes the excretion of the following drugs:

- a Tricyclic antidepressants
- b Barbiturates
- c Amphetamine
- d Atropine
- e Pethidine

27 Intravenous administration of histamine can cause:

- a Increased gastric secretion
- b Headache
- c Intestinal colic
- d Tachycardia
- e Increased airway resistance

28 Antisialogogue drugs:

- a Act on the muscarinic receptors of acetylcholine
- b May produce bronchodilation
- c All cross the placenta
- d May produce amnesia
- e Increase lower oesophageal sphincter tone

29 Enzyme induction is seen with the following:

- a Phenylbutazone
- b Phenytoin
- c Cimetidine
- d Phenobarbital (phenobarbitone)
- e Etomidate

30 Phenothiazines:

a Have a three-ringed structure
b Have no effect on the CTZ
c Have an alpha blocking action
d Fluorine substitution at positions 2 and 10 increases their potency
e Have an antimuscarinic action

chapter 1 PHARMACOLOGY

ANSWERS

1 Suxamethonium:

a **True** It is a dicholine ester of succinic acid. It is effectively two acetylcholine molecules joined back to back through their acetyl groups.

b **True** Quaternary ammonium groups make it a highly charged compound, thus making it non-permeable to lipid membranes, mainly the blood–brain barrier.

c **False** Suxamethonium is one of the drugs causing significant histamine release. This is apparent predominantly in the upper torso and face as flushing developing soon after injection.

d **True** Patients with abnormal genes coding for plasma cholinesterase will have prolonged neuromuscular block and can be treated with fresh frozen plasma (FFP) providing a source of plasma cholinesterase or they may be sedated and ventilated until the block wears off.

e **False** Suxamethonium on its own without any inhalational agent can trigger malignant hyperpyrexia.

Table 1.1 Side effects of suxamethonium

Side effect	Mechanism
Bradycardia	Probably via mAChR in the heart; mainly seen in children; opposed by atropine
Myalgia	Most common in young ambulatory female patients; worse in the shoulder and pelvic girdle muscles; caused by muscle damage secondary to fasiculations
Increased intragastric pressure	Thought to be due to abdominal muscle fasiculations; no increased risk of regurgitation as lower oesophageal sphincter tone is also increased (unless this mechanism is altered, e.g. pregnancy)
Increased intracranial and intraocular pressure	Transient rise after injection—of no importance unless there is eye or intracranial pathology: in such cases, the risk–benefit balance should be carefully considered and suxamethonium avoided if possible.
Hyperkalaemia	Usually by 0.5mmol/l but higher in certain conditions (see below) when it should be avoided if possible
Hypotension	Caused by muscle relaxation, bradycardia, and histamine release
Tachyphylaxis	Repeated doses may cause a reduced response and lead to a change to phase 2 block (similar to NDMRs); more likely with large doses and infusions (rarely used)
Anaphylaxis	Ranging from minor skin flushing to severe bronchospasm and cardiac arrest
Suxamethonium apnoea	Due to acquired or genetic factors
Malignant hyperpyrexia	Suxamethonium is a potent trigger for malignant hyperthermia

mAChR, muscarinic acetylcholine receptor; NDMR, non-depolarizing muscle relaxant.

Kevin K and Spoors C (2009) *Training in Anaesthesia*. New York: Oxford University Press.
Rang H, Dale M, and Ritter J (2000) *Rang and Dales' Pharmacology*, 6th edition. Edinburgh: Churchill Livingstone.

2 Morphine:

a **True** Nitrous oxide has been used as an analgesic on its own in various situations including physiotherapy and dressing changes, and has been said to provide equipotent analgesia to 15 mg of morphine.

b **False** Morphine stimulates ADH secretion significantly, and may lead to impaired water excretion and hyponatraemia.

c **True** Morphine may cause spasm of the sphincter of Oddi, although this is rarely a significant problem. Previously an anticholinergic such as atropine was co-administered to prevent this.

d **True** Acute trauma may induce gastric stasis and administration of morphine will depress gastric motility further. This should be remembered when anaesthetizing trauma patients.

e **False** Morphine stimulates the CTZ via 5-hydroxytryptamine$_3$ ($5HT_3$) and dopamine receptors.

Aitkenhead A and Smith G (2008) *Textbook of Anaesthesia*, 5th edition. Edinburgh: Churchill Livingstone.

3 Ranitidine:

a **False** It is an H_2 receptor antagonist, like cimetidine.

b **True** The pH is increased and the volume of secretions is decreased. It is used in high-risk labouring women for these actions. It does not have an effect on gastric motility.

c **False** The intravenous dose is 50 mg. It should be diluted to 20 ml and injected slowly to prevent bradycardia. The oral dose is 150 mg.

d **False** Cimetidine inhibits hepatic cytochrome P450, however ranitidine does not. The latter is also more potent, making it a more popular H_2 antagonist.

e **True** It may precipitate an attack in porphyric patients.

Allman K and Wilson I (2006) *Oxford Handbook of Anaesthesia*, 2nd edition. New York: Oxford University Press.

4 Regarding ultra-short-acting barbiturates:

a **True** Malonic acid plus urea produce malonyl urea, which is the primary molecule of a barbiturate.

b **False** They are metabolized slowly in the liver (half-life 8.4 hours) before being renally excreted.

c **True** Evidence suggests that they have a protective action on the brain and have previously been used for this purpose in intensive care.

d **False** Their solubility depends on transformation from keto to enol form, which occurs more readily in alkaline solutions.

e **True** Barbiturates are better excreted by alkalinizing the urine.

Rang H, Dale M, and Ritter J (2000) *Rang and Dales' Pharmacology*, 6th edition. Edinburgh: Churchill Livingstone.

5 Hydantoin derivatives:

- a **True** Hydantoin derivatives, e.g. phenytoin and fosphenytoin, have been used in the treatment of epilepsy along with barbiturates.
- b **True** They bind and stabilize inactivated sodium channels preventing action potential generation and therefore seizure activity.
- c **True** CNS depression occurs with the membrane-stabilizing effect; in addition calcium entry into neurones is prevented, which further prevents neurotransmitter release and potentiates the actions of gamma-aminobutyric acid (GABA).
- d **True** They have been used in the treatment of certain dysrhythmias. Phenytoin is a class 1b antiarrhythmic drug that is useful in treating ventricular dysrhythmias.
- e **True** Dantrolene is a hydantoin derivative.

Rang H, Dale M, and Ritter J (2000) *Rang and Dales' Pharmacology*, 6th edition. Edinburgh: Churchill Livingstone.

6 Diuretic therapy leads to:

- a **False** Thiazide diuretics produce hypochloraemic alkalosis as well as hyponatraemia, hypokalaemia, and hypermagnesaemia.
- b **False** These drugs produce metabolic acidosis. Carbonic anhydrase inhibitors are still used topically to treat glaucoma. They can be also used as a simple method of treating metabolic alkalosis in the acute clinical situation and in counteracting the respiratory alkalosis in altitude sickness.
- c **True** Symptoms in patients with gout are exacerbated if they are simultaneously treated with thiazide diuretics.
- d **True** Hyperglycaemia is seen with the loop diuretics, although not as commonly as with thiazides. Closer blood sugar monitoring is required for diabetic patients taking these diuretics.
- e **False** This is a potassium-sparing diuretic which is often used with loop diuretics to prevent hypokalaemia.

Peck T, Hill S, and Williams M (2004) *Pharmacology for Anaesthesia and Intensive Care*, 2nd edition. Cambridge: Cambridge University Press.

7 Cocaine:

- a **False** It was the first ester derived from the leaves of the plant *Erythroxylon coca*. Sigmund Freud treated a morphine addict by substituting it with cocaine. The patient complained of a numb mouth, prompting Freud to suggest to his ophthalmologist friend Karl Koller to try it as a surface anaesthetic for eye surgery.
- b **True** Its first documented use was when Karl Koller used it for ophthalmic surgery in 1884.
- c **True** It produces topical anaesthesia and local vasoconstriction, thus making it useful when administered nasally for ENT surgery.
- d **True** Cocaine causes vasoconstriction and can produce hyperthermia.
- e **True** Cocaine inhibits 'uptake 1' and monoamine oxidase, stimulating the sympathetic nervous system.

Allman K and Wilson I (2006) *Oxford Handbook of Anaesthesia*, 2nd edition. USA: Oxford University Press.

8 Thiopental (thiopentone):

a **False** The pH of 2.5% thiopental has been quoted as being between 10.8 and 11.
b **True** Thiopental is the sulphur analogue of the oxybarbiturate pentobarbitone.
c **True** Over 80% is protein bound. Despite this it has a rapid onset due to high lipid solubility and the large cardiac output that the brain receives.
d **False** At two minutes post induction most of the drug is in the vessel-rich group of organs, at four minutes the major portion (>80%) is in the muscles, and at about seven minutes it reaches the fatty tissue. The drug recirculates slowly (half-life 8.4 hours) and is metabolized in the liver before being excreted renally.
e **True** In porphyria, thiopental can produce a syndrome that resembles a demyelination state.

Rang H, Dale M, and Ritter J (2000) *Rang and Dales' Pharmacology*, 6th edition. Edinburgh: Churchill Livingstone.

9 The following are potassium-sparing diuretics:

a **False** It is a carbonic anhydrase inhibitor that increases sodium and potassium excretion and reduces water absorption.
b **False** Furosemide and other loop diuretics inhibit sodium and chloride reabsorption in the thick ascending loop of Henle and early distal convoluted tubule leading to reduced water reabsorption. They cause hyponatraemia, hypokalaemia, and hypomagnesaemia, and can produce hypochloraemic alkalosis.
c **False** Thiazide diuretics inhibit sodium and chloride reabsorption in the early distal convoluted tubule thus promoting increased water excretion. The increased sodium load in the distal tubule is exchanged for potassium and hydrogen ions thus producing a hypokalaemic hypochloraemic alkalosis.
d **True** Spironolactone is a competitive aldosterone antagonist. Therefore in the distal tubule potassium excretion is reduced and sodium excretion is increased producing the diuretic effect.
e **True** Amiloride acts independently of aldosterone at the distal convoluted tubule blocking sodium/potassium exchange, conserving potassium and producing diuresis.

Table 1.2 Actions of diuretics

	Na^+ excretion (%)	K^+ excretion	Bicarbonate excretion	Ca^{2+} excretion	Free water excretion
Osmotic	10	↑	↑	↑	↑
CAI	5–10	↑	↑	↑	↑
Loop	25	↑	↓	↓	↓
Thiazide	5–10	↑	↓	↓	↓
Potassium-sparing	3–5	↓	↑	NA	NA
Aquaretic	0	NA	NA	NA	↑

CAI, carbonic anhydrase inhibitor.

Kevin K and Spoors C (2009) *Training in Anaesthesia*. USA: Oxford University Press.
Peck T, Hill S, and Williams M (2004) *Pharmacology for Anaesthesia and Intensive Care*, 2nd edition. Cambridge: Cambridge University Press.

10 Regarding local anaesthetic drugs:

a **True** The trachea is more vascular and therefore absorption is quicker.

b **False** Local anaesthetic drugs work more efficiently in an alkaline medium than the acidic medium of an infected site. This is because the acidic environment reduces the un-ionized fraction of the drug available to diffuse into the nerve and block it.

c **True** Although this is true regarding prilocaine, it is not a common occurrence. It is suggested that following high doses of lidocaine (lignocaine) similar findings may be seen.

d **False** 8% dextrose is added to bupivacaine 0.5% to produce heavy bupivacaine. This is the only additive licensed for subarachnoid use and other preservatives are not added as they pose a risk of arachnoiditis.

e **True** Dibucaine is an amide local anaesthetic that inhibits normal plasma cholinesterase. It inhibits the variant forms of plasma cholinesterase less effectively. Dibucaine inhibits the normal form by 80% and other forms by 20–80%, depending on the type involved. The percentage inhibition is known as the 'dibucaine number'. This number represents the genotype of the individual but does not quantify the enzyme in the plasma.

Peck T, Hill S, and Williams M (2004) *Pharmacology for Anaesthesia and Intensive Care*, 2nd edition. Cambridge: Cambridge University Press.

11 The following drugs reduce afterload:

a **True** Aminophylline is mainly used as a bronchodilator. Care is required during its IV administration because of the significant fall in afterload causing severe hypotension. When given slowly it has an inotropic action.

b **False** Because it has effects on both alpha and beta receptors it may cause a rise in the afterload because of the beta action. Hence it is suggested that it is better to use a drug for altering the alpha effects first before administering the beta blocker.

c **False** It primarily produces venodilation and reduces the preload preferentially.

d **True** Isoprenaline being a pure beta agonist reduces the afterload as well being an inotropic agent.

e **False** Noradrenaline (norepinephrine) increases the total peripheral resistance thereby increasing the afterload.

Peck T, Hill S, and Williams M (2004) *Pharmacology for Anaesthesia and Intensive Care*, 2nd edition. Cambridge: Cambridge University Press.

12 The following are examples of competitive antagonism:

a **True** These compete for the same receptor site at the neuromuscular junction.

b **False** No direct interaction exists with salicylates and oral hypoglycaemics.

c **False** The enzyme induction with barbiturates increases the metabolism of anticoagulant drugs necessitating higher dosage of the latter. When barbiturate intake is stopped there could be a life-threatening bleeding tendency if a coagulation screen is not undertaken promptly and the anticoagulant dose reduced.

d **True** They compete for the same opioid receptor.

e **True** Chlorpromazine has both a central and peripheral action. Peripherally it would be a dopaminergic receptor blocker.

Rang H, Dale M, and Ritter J (2000) *Rang and Dales' Pharmacology*, 6th edition. Edinburgh: Churchill Livingstone.

13 Administration of the following may reduce renal blood flow:

a **False** Xanthines have a diuretic effect due to a direct action on renal tubules but do not reduce blood flow.

b **False** Ephedrine has both alpha and beta activity but it is not potent enough to affect renal blood flow.

c **True** This inhalational agent is no longer used; it actively stimulated ADH secretion and reduced hepatic and renal blood flow.

d **False** Isoprenaline is pure beta stimulant and does not interfere with renal blood flow.

e **False** Dobutamine actively increases urinary output by improving cardiac output, but does not alter renal blood flow.

Peck T, Hill S, and Williams M (2004) *Pharmacology for Anaesthesia and Intensive Care*, 2nd edition. Cambridge: Cambridge University Press.

14 Remifentanil:

a **True** It acts rapidly and the action is terminated quickly after discontinuation of the infusion.

b **False** It is hydrolysed by non-specific esterases.

c **False** The effect lasts for 5–10 minutes.

d **True** Like all other synthetic opioids, remifentanil can induce muscle rigidity.

e **True** Remifentanil has been used for analgesia in labour, however, a high incidence of respiratory depression limits its widespread use.

Allman K and Wilson I (2006) *Oxford Handbook of Anaesthesia*, 2nd edition. New York: Oxford University Press.

15 Nicotinic actions of acetylcholine include:

a **False** Salivation is mediated by muscarinic receptors.

b **False** Bronchospasm is mediated by muscarinic receptors. Antimuscarinic agents are used in the treatment of asthma.

c **False** Bradycardia is mediated by muscarinic receptors.

d **True** Acetylcholine stimulates nicotinic receptors at the postsynaptic neuromuscular junction.

e **True** It has effects on neural transmission in the ascending pathways to the cortex and the basal ganglia, causing initial CNS stimulation followed by depression.

Yentis S, Hirsh N, and Smith G (2003) *Anaesthesia and Intensive Care A to Z*, 3rd edition. London: Butterworth-Heinemann.

16 Isoflurane:

a **False** The boiling point of isoflurane is 49°C.

b **False** The MAC of isoflurane 1.17. Halothane has a MAC of 0.75.

c **False** Very little isoflurane is metabolized, only 0.2%. Trifluoroacetic acid is a metabolite of halothane. The 'rule of 2' shows the metabolism of desflurane, isoflurane, enflurane, and halothane to be 0.02%, 0.2%, 2%, and 20%, respectively.

d **True** Isoflurane has a saturated vapour pressure of 33 kPa.

e **False** Thymol was a preservative used as a stabilizing agent in the storage of halothane.

Peck T, Hill S, and Williams M (2004) *Pharmacology for Anaesthesia and Intensive Care*, 2nd edition. Cambridge: Cambridge University Press.

17 Therapeutic excess of oral anticoagulants may be reversed with:

a **False** Aprotinin acts as an antifibrinolytic agent.
b **True** Vitamin K is the specific antagonist. Care should be taken not to use a high dose of vitamin K, which may induce a hypercoagulable state.
c **False** HAS contains albumin suspended in saline. It has no clotting factors.
d **True** FFP contains all the clotting factors.
e **True** Cryoprecipitate is very effective on its own or in combination with vitamin K.

Aitkenhead A and Smith G (2008) *Textbook of Anaesthesia*, 5th edition. Edinburgh: Churchill Livingstone.

18 Ganglionic blocking drugs produce:

a **True** Trimetaphan is an example which was used intraoperatively to produce controlled hypotension until newer drugs such as labetalol and sodium nitroprusside became readily available.
b **False** Mydriasis that persists for a considerable time is the usual response. Recovery staff had to be specifically warned about this when trimetaphan was used in order to prevent mistaken assumptions of an cerebral event on account of the dilated pupils.
c **False** The parasympathetic blockade produced would cause decreased intestinal motility.
d **False** Compensatory tachycardia is the usual response.
e **False** Sweating is reduced.

Ganglion blockers competitively antagonize nicotinic receptors at both parasympathetic and sympathetic ganglia, and the adrenal cortex. They have a direct vasodilator effect on peripheral vessels.

Peck T, Hill S, and Williams M (2004) *Pharmacology for Anaesthesia and Intensive Care*, 2nd edition. Cambridge: Cambridge University Press.

19 Drugs used in the diagnosis or treatment of myasthenia gravis include:

a **True** The 'Tensilon test' as it is known, helps differentiate between a myasthenic and a cholinergic crisis. Edrophonium is given IV, and improvement in muscle strength indicates a myasthenic crisis whereas worsening of weakness is seen in cholinergic crisis.
b **False** Pralidoxime is a reactivator of acetylcholinesterase used in the treatment of organophosphate poisoning.
c **False** Amantadine is a drug used in treatment of Parkinson's disease.
d **False** Decamethonium was a depolarizing neuromuscular blocking drug used in the past.
e **False** Aminopyridine was previously used to reverse non-depolarizing neuromuscular blockade and to treat myasthenic syndrome (Eaton–Lambert syndrome). It did not inhibit acetylcholinesterase but acted presynaptically to increase acetylcholine release and increase the force of muscle contraction.

Table 1.3 Comparison of acetylcholinesterase inhibitors

	Name	Neostigmine	Pyridostigmine	Edrophonium
Properties	Uses	For reversal of NDMRs; MG therapy	Main use in MG; Can be used to reverse NDMR block	Tensilon test For reversal of NDMRs
	Chemical	Quaternary amine	Pyridine analogue of neostigmine	Synthetic quaternary ammonium compound
	Presentation	Clear colourless solution for IV injection	Clear colourless solution for IV injection 5 mg/ml	Clear colourless solution, 10 mg/ml
	Action	Cholinergic	Cholinergic; fewer muscarinic effects than neostigmine	Cholinergic
	Mode	Reversible acid-transferring cholinesterase inhibitor; binds to the esteratic site	Reversible acid-transferring cholinesterase inhibitor; binds to the esteratic site	Competes with ACh at the anionic site of cholinesterase; some pre-junctional action
	Route	MG dose: 15–50 mg 2–4 hrly Reversal: 0.05 mg/kg, with anticholinergic agent	IV, IM, or PO for MG; 60 mg tablets; dose titrated to effect	IV administration; more rapid onset and briefer duration than neostig-mine
Effects	CVS	↓HR and ↓CO, ↑conduction time, ↓ refractory period.	Slower onset ↓HR and ↓CO; ↑conduction time and ↓refractory period	↓HR, ↓CO; ↑conduction time
	RS	↑secretion, bronchoconstriction	↑secretion, bronchoconstriction	↑secretion, broncho-constriction
	CNS	High doses: causes neuromuscular blockade by direct receptor effects and accumulation of ACh	High doses: causes blockade by direct effect and accumulation of ACh	Agitation, miosis; weakness and fascicula-tion in normal subjects
	GI	↑salivation, ↑gastric secretions, ↑motility	↑salivation, ↑gastric secretions, ↑motility	↑salivation, ↑GI motility, ↑gastric acid secretions
	Other	↑ureteric peristalsis	↑ureteric peristalsis	↑ureteric peristalsis
Kinetics	Absorption	Poor oral absorption; 1–2% oral bioavailability	<10% oral bioavailability	
	Distribution	Highly ionized; 6–10% protein bound		V_D 0.9–1.3 l/kg
	Metabolism	Metabolized to quaternary alcohol by plasma estera-ses; some biliary excretion	<25% metabolized and subsequently glucuronidated	Uncertain; it is not hydrolysed by esterases
	Excretion	66% excreted in the urine; renal failure leads to accumulation	Renal excretion accounts for 75% of clearance	Unknown
	Notes	Prolongs action of suxamethonium	Longer to peak effect than neostigmine	Cardiac arrest has been reported

CVS, cardiovascular system; GI, gastrointestinal; RS, respiratory system; MG, myasthenia gravis; HR, heart rate; CO, cardiac output; ACh, acetyl choline; IM, intramuscular; PO, peroral; V_D, volume distribution; NDMR, non-depolarizing muscle relaxant.

Peck T, Hill S, and Williams M (2004) *Pharmacology for Anaesthesia and Intensive Care*, 2nd edition. Cambridge: Cambridge University Press.
Yentis S, Hirsh N, and Smith G (2003) *Anaesthesia and Intensive Care A to Z*, 3rd edition. London: Butterworth-Heinemann.

20 Glycopyrrolate:

a **False** Glycopyrrolate being a quaternary ammonium compound is charged and does not cross the blood–brain barrier. Therefore it is devoid of central effects. Hyoscine does cross the blood–brain barrier, producing significant sedation, and was previously employed as premedication for this effect.

b **True** 500 μg is added to 2.5 mg of neostigmine in an ampoule designed to reverse neuromuscular blockade in an adult.

c **False** Glycopyrrolate does not have a significant effect on intraocular pressure unlike atropine, which increases intraocular pressure when applied topically.

d **True** Glycopyrrolate may be used in children. It is occasionally used as a premedication for its antisialogogue effects.

e **True** Unlike atropine, which has been known to produce ventricular ectopics, glycopyrrolate is known to produce supraventricular ectopic beats occasionally.

Peck T, Hill S, and Williams M (2004) *Pharmacology for Anaesthesia and Intensive Care*, 2nd edition. Cambridge: Cambridge University Press.

21 Derivatives of opium include:

a **False** It is a synthetic opioid used in the management of addiction to opiates. It has a longer duration of action than morphine and diamorphine and has less of a euphoric effect. It is occasionally used in the treatment of chronic pain.

b **False** Pethidine is a synthetic opioid and is licensed to be administered by midwives without a doctor's prescription.

c **False** Dextropropoxyphene is another opioid which in combination with paracetamol used to be prescribed as 'Distalgesic' tablets in the perioperative period. It is no longer available.

d **True** Codeine is one of the alkaloids of opium.

e **True** Papaveretum is a crude extract of opium and was very popular until the 1990s. It contained morphine, codeine and papaverine.

Peck T, Hill S, and Williams M (2004) *Pharmacology for Anaesthesia and Intensive Care*, 2nd edition. Cambridge: Cambridge University Press.
Rang H, Dale M, and Ritter J (2000) *Rang and Dales' Pharmacology*, 6th edition. Edinburgh: Churchill Livingstone.

22 Cyanide poisoning:

a **False** Glyceryl trinitrate is not implicated in cyanide formation, but sodium nitroprusside is.

b **False** Since the tissues are incapable of accepting oxygen, the venous blood remains saturated and the arterio-venous difference is therefore decreased.

c **False** Oxygen partial pressure is not affected.

d **False** Arterial pH tends to decrease after a while.

e **True** Methylene blue has been suggested as one therapy in conjunction with others.

Peck T, Hill S, and Williams M (2004) *Pharmacology for Anaesthesia and Intensive Care*, 2nd edition. Cambridge: Cambridge University Press.
Yentis S, Hirsh N, and Smith G (2003) *Anaesthesia and Intensive Care A to Z*, 3rd edition. London: Butterworth-Heinemann.

23 Drugs producing bronchodilation include:

a **True** Aminophylline is a xanthine derivative.
b **False** Muscarine produces bronchospasm.
c **False** Pilocarpine has a similar cholinergic action to muscarine producing bronchospasm.
d **False** 5HT has a similar action to histamine, producing bronchospasm.
e **True** Diethyl ether was a potent bronchodilator among inhalational agents. Although it was irritant if a high dose was administered suddenly, a slow induction with ether made the agent acceptable and caused bronchodilation.

Rang H, Dale M, and Ritter J (2000) *Rang and Dales' Pharmacology*, 6th edition. Edinburgh: Churchill Livingstone.

24 Adverse effects of nitrous oxide include:

a **True** Nitrous oxide trapped in the middle ear can lead to transient deafness.
b **True** Long-term use produces agranulocytosis and marrow aplasia.
c **True** This is a well-known phenomenon immediately post anaesthesia if supplemental oxygen is not administered.
d **True** Nitric or nitrous oxide can produce nitric acid and pulmonary oedema.
e **False** Cranial nerve palsy has not been linked to nitrous oxide.

Rang H, Dale M, and Ritter J (2000) *Rang and Dales' Pharmacology*, 6th edition. Edinburgh: Churchill Livingstone.

25 Induction is more rapid with an inhalational agent:

a **True** The lower the blood/gas partition coefficient the faster the induction.
b **False** The oil/gas partition coefficient determines the potency of the agent and not the speed of induction.
c **True** Hyperventilation caused by carbon dioxide increases the delivery of inhalational agent to the alveolus, increasing the alveolar tension and therefore the equilibration with the brain tension producing a more rapid onset of anaesthesia.
d **True** More of the agent can be supplied quickly.
e **True** With the ability to give a high concentration of sevoflurane, the lower cardiac output in the elderly means that the tension in the alveolus is able to build up more rapidly, thus increasing the tension in the brain. With traditional inhalational agents, however, incremental increases in concentration were required, and with altered respiratory physiology in the elderly made induction with these agents much slower than in younger subjects.

Aitkenhead A and Smith G. (2008) *Textbook of Anaesthesia*, 5th edition. Edinburgh: Churchill Livingstone.

26 Alkaline diuresis promotes the excretion of the following drugs:

a **False** Management is largely supportive. Although induction of alkalaemia (pH>7.5) is used to reduce the amount of free drug forced alkaline diuresis is not used.
b **True** Salicylates and barbiturates are effectively cleared with forced alkaline diuresis although availability of haemofiltration means this technique is rarely used now.
c **False** Amphetamines can be cleared by an acid diuresis.
d **False** Alkaline diuresis will not aid excretion of atropine. Anticholinesterase drugs such as physostigmine will counteract the CNS and cardiovascular effects of atropine poisoning.
e **False** Pethidine is cleared with acid diuresis.

Aitkenhead A and Smith G (2008) *Textbook of Anaesthesia*, 5th edition. Edinburgh: Churchill Livingstone.

27 IV administration of histamine can cause:

a **True** Histamine acts on H_2 receptors causing increased acid, pepsin and intrinsic factor secretion from the gastric mucosa.
b **True** Vasodilation can lead to headache mediated via H_1 and H_2 receptors.
c **True** H_1-mediated smooth muscle contraction in the gastrointestinal tract can cause symptoms of colic.
d **True** A H_2-related increase in heart rate occurs.
e **True** H_1-mediated bronchoconstriction occurs and via stimulation of irritant pulmonary receptors.

Yentis S, Hirsh N, and Smith G (2003) *Anaesthesia and Intensive Care A to Z*, 3rd edition. London: Butterworth-Heinemann.

28 Antisialogogue drugs:

a **True** They act on the muscarinic receptors of acetylcholine. They are termed 'anticholinergics' but at normal doses are entirely antimuscarinic.
b **True** Atropine and glycopyrrolate cause more bronchodilation than hyoscine.
c **False** Both atropine and hyoscine are naturally occurring tertiary amines and are able to cross the placenta and blood–brain barrier. Glycopyrrolate, however, is a quaternary amine, i.e. charged and is therefore unable to cross the placenta or blood–brain barrier.
d **True** Atropine and hyoscine can cross the blood–brain barrier causing central effects. Hyoscine produces amnesia and was used in premedication for this effect. Glycopyrrolate exhibits no central effects as it does not cross the blood–brain barrier.
e **False** They decrease the tone of the lower oesophageal sphincter.

Peck T, Hill S, and Williams M (2004) *Pharmacology for Anaesthesia and Intensive Care*, 2nd edition. Cambridge: Cambridge University Press.

29 Enzyme induction may be seen with the following drugs:

a **False** Phenylbutazone is an extremely potent anti-inflammatory, only licensed for use in inpatients under specialist supervision due to its serious haematological side effects. It reduces hepatic function.
b **True** Phenytoin causes hepatic enzyme induction. It induces its own metabolism.
c **False** Cimetidine is an enzyme inhibitor and reduces metabolism of lidocaine, labetalol, propranolol, nifedipine, warfarin, phenytoin, and theophylline. It has therefore been superseded by ranitidine, which is more potent and does not inhibit hepatic enzymes.
d **True** The most potent enzyme inducer, first noticed for the sudden rise in bleeding tendency when inpatients (who were on long-term phenobarbital and warfarin) were discharged without sedatives, thus leading to overdose of warfarin.
e **False** Etomidate is an enzyme inhibitor. Etomidate leads to adrenocortical suppression and has produced fatal outcomes when administered by infusion in intensive care. Following these deaths, legislation now requires that to license a new drug for continuous infusion, it should be proved conclusively and beyond doubt that the drug does not interfere with adrenal cortical function.

Peck T, Hill S, and Williams M (2004) *Pharmacology for Anaesthesia and Intensive Care*, 2nd edition. Cambridge: Cambridge University Press.
Rang H, Dale M, and Ritter J (2000) *Rang and Dales' Pharmacology*, 6th edition. Edinburgh: Churchill Livingstone.

30 Phenothiazines:

a **True** The side chains confer different pharmacological characteristics.

b **False** They have antiemetic properties, hence have an effect on the CTZ.

c **True** Chlorpromazine has a strong alpha blocking action producing vasodilation, hypotension, and heat loss.

d **True** By fluorine substitution at these two sites, phenothiazines become better antipsychotic and better antiemetic drugs.

e **True** They are antimuscarinic, producing bronchodilation.

Peck T, Hill S, and Williams M (2004) *Pharmacology for Anaesthesia and Intensive Care*, 2nd edition. Cambridge: Cambridge University Press.

Rang H, Dale M, and Ritter J (2000) *Rang and Dales' Pharmacology*, 6th edition. Edinburgh: Churchill Livingstone.

chapter 1

PHYSICS

QUESTIONS

1 Rotameters:

- a Are variable orifice flow meters
- b Contain bobbins that denote the actual flow rate
- c Are non-linear in their calibration
- d Exhibit a turbulent flow pattern at low gas flows
- e Deliver approximately 40 l/min of oxygen if the bobbin is left at the very top

2 Regarding gases:

- a Pressure in a cylinder of Entonox® is 137 bar
- b Boyle's law relates gas volume to temperature at constant pressure
- c Flow in the terminal airways is essentially turbulent
- d Kinematic viscosity is the ratio of the viscosity of a fluid to its density at which point flow becomes turbulent
- e The stoichiometric concentration is the concentration at which all the combustible vapour and oxidizing agent are completely used up

3 Nitrogen:

- a Has a lower boiling point than oxygen
- b Diffuses faster than carbon dioxide
- c Is used in the storage of certain drugs by the pharmaceutical industry
- d Is employed as a drying agent for new or tested cylinders
- e Under increased ambient pressure may produce narcosis

4 Oxygen:

- a Can be manufactured by heating barium oxide to 800°C
- b Manufacture uses the principle of adiabatic expansion during fractional distillation of air
- c Is supplied in cylinders at a pressure of 180 kPa
- d Diffuses more rapidly from the alveolus than nitrous oxide
- e Tension in the blood can be measured by oximetry

5 A wet spirometer can be used to directly measure:

- a Tidal volume
- b Inspiratory capacity
- c Oxygen consumption per minute
- d Functional residual capacity
- e Vital capacity

6 Oxygen delivery systems:

- a Nasal cannulae are capable of delivering a fraction of inspired oxygen (FiO_2) of 60% at oxygen flow rates of 4–6 l/min
- b High flow, air entrainment masks are the most efficient devices
- c Ventimasks have a Venturi system with a fixed 8:1 ratio for entrainment of air
- d To minimize rebreathing and deliver a fixed concentration of oxygen, the flow rate should match the maximum inspiratory flow rate of the patient
- e To reliably deliver 100% oxygen the 'Mapleson A' circuit should be used

7 Regarding humidification:

- a Approximately 28 mg of water per litre has to be added to the room air at 20°C temperature to produce a saturated vapour pressure(SVP) of 47 mmHg in the alveolus
- b 'Dew point' is the term used when the relative humidity reaches 100% at a given temperature
- c Particle size is of paramount importance for efficient humidification of the terminal airways
- d Ultrasonic nebulizers function at around 1.5 MHz
- e The 'Bernoulli effect' is the principle behind air entrainment devices

8 Cardiac output can be measured by:

- a Dye dilution techniques
- b Thermal dilution techniques
- c Impedance plethysmography
- d Body plethysmography
- e Ballistocardiography

9 Oxygen analysis can be performed using the following apparatus:

- a Clark electrode
- b Van Slyke apparatus
- c Daniel cell
- d Fuel cell
- e Weston cell

10 The Vitalograph:

- a Is a specialized dry spirometer
- b Provides the gas volume readings corrected to body temperature (37°C) and pressure (atmospheric), saturated (47 mmHg) (BTPS) on one side of the chart
- c Is used for measuring forced expiratory volume in one second (FEV_1)
- d Can be used for measuring peak expiratory flow rate (PEFR)
- e Can be used for estimation of maximum voluntary ventilation (MVV)

11 Infrared analysers can be used for the estimation of:

- a Carbon dioxide
- b Nitrous oxide
- c Isoflurane
- d Halothane
- e Oxygen

12 PEEP:

a Is the acronym for positive end-expiratory pressure
b Is applied with a PEEP valve positioned at the expiratory limb of the ventilator circuit
c Valves can achieve a pressure of 0–20 cmH_2O
d Is responsible for barotrauma at the higher range of pressures
e Is useful in improving oxygenation, but delivery of oxygen may be reduced because of lower cardiac output

13 The following are examples of pressure release devices:

a Bourdon gauge
b Aneroid gauge
c Ruben valve
d Heidbrink valve
e Frumen valve

14 Soda lime:

a Consists of a combination of 60% sodium hydroxide and 35% calcium hydroxide granules
b Should be of 2–3 mesh size to function efficiently
c Can be used in a 'Mapleson C' circuit
d May form carbon monoxide if inhalational agents are passed over it when it is desiccated
e Has been implicated in cranial nerve palsy in the past when the temperature inside the canister had reached over 60°C during use

15 A transducer:

a Is a device that converts mechanical energy into electrical energy
b May be applied to inaccessible sites in the body
c Using the Wheatstone bridge principle is employed for blood pressure monitoring
d Using the photoelectric cell principle, converts light waves to an electrical signal
e Should possess a resonant frequency greater than the oscillations to which it is responding.

16 Vaporizers:

a Employ the Plenum principle
b Tec Mark 3 and later models are capable of maintaining a steady output between 18°C and 36°C
c Contain steel wicks in the vaporizing chamber
d Need not be recalibrated for use in a hyperbaric chamber
e Are very efficient for use as a vaporizer inside the circuit (VIC)

17 During anaesthesia under hyperbaric conditions:

a Nitrous oxide should always be used to reduce risk of explosion
b Reducing valves need to be changed
c Flow meters may read higher than the flow being delivered
d Endotracheal cuffs should be inflated with water
e Only infusions contained in glass bottles should be used

18 The following may be used for sterilization of equipment:

- a Formaldehyde
- b Infrared radiation
- c Gamma radiation
- d Ethanol
- e Ethylene glycol

19 The hot air oven is not as efficient as an autoclave because:

- a Dry heat has to be applied for longer periods at higher temperatures
- b 1 litre of air cooling from 160°C to 150°C gives off only 0.2 cal compared with 1 litre of steam giving out 870 cal of heat at a constant temperature of 134°C
- c Dry heat penetrates only by direct conduction
- d Dry heat kills by coagulation whereas moist heat kills by oxidation of protein
- e The thermal death point of microorganisms is lower when exposed to wet rather than dry heat

20 Concerning the gas laws:

- a Boyle's law relates volume of gas to temperature at a constant pressure
- b Dalton's law relates to the total pressure exerted by a mixture of gases as being the arithmetic sum of their individual pressures
- c Henry's law is concerned with diffusion of gases across a membrane
- d Gay Lussac's law relates pressure of a gas to temperature at constant volume
- e Charles' law relates the pressure of a gas to the volume at constant temperature

21 The following gases are lighter than air:

- a Nitrous oxide
- b Cyclopropane
- c Carbon dioxide
- d Diethyl ether
- e Ethylene oxide

22 Concerning flow of a gas or liquid through a tube:

- a Resistance is directly proportional to the viscosity
- b Flow is directly proportional to the square of density
- c Resistance is inversely proportional to the square of the radius
- d Critical velocity is the flow velocity at which energy loss occurs between the layers of fluid
- e During turbulent flow, the flow rate is directly proportional to the square root of the pressure drop

23 In statistical terms:

- a Any observation recorded is a variable
- b The commonest measure of central tendency is the mean
- c Degrees of freedom is equal to the number in the sample
- d The most commonly occurring value is the mode
- e The value of the middle observation is the variance

24 Statistical tests of significance include:

a Student's 't' test
b Wilcoxon's two-sample rank sum test
c Sequential analysis
d Chi-squared test
e Regression analysis

25 The apparatus given below has the following uses:

a Oximeter measuring partial pressure of oxygen
b Pneumotachograph measuring airway resistance
c Impedance plethysmograph measuring lung volumes
d Flame photometer measuring serum calcium
e Katharometer measuring potential difference across an electrical circuit

26 Doppler-shift instruments are used for:

a Measurement of blood flow
b Measurement of arterial pressure
c Detection of air emboli
d Apnoea monitors
e Estimation of cardiac output

27 Regarding radiation:

a The atomic number is equal to the number of protons in the atom
b Isotopes are atoms with the same number of protons but extra electrons
c The biological half-life of a radioactive isotope is the same as the physical half-life
d Ionizing radiation is used for sterilizing disposable anaesthetic equipment in the manufacturing process
e A Geiger counter is normally employed to detect free radiation

28 For ventilating a patient with high airway resistance:

a A constant pressure ventilator should be used
b Tidal volume should be increased
c Inspiratory flow rate should be increased
d Respiratory rate should be increased
e Negative end-expiratory pressure (NEEP) should be employed

29 Anaesthetic breathing circuits:

a The 'Mapleson D' circuit is the most efficient for controlled ventilation
b 'Mapleson B' has been used for paediatric anaesthesia
c The 'Lack' circuit requires a flow rate of twice the minute volume for spontaneous ventilation
d Jackson Rees modified the 'Mapleson C' circuit
e The resistance of the expiratory valve should not be more than 2–3 cmH_2O during spontaneous ventilation

30 Entonox®:

a Is manufactured by bubbling oxygen through an inverted cylinder containing nitrous oxide in liquid form

b The process of mixing nitrous oxide and oxygen is known as the 'Poynting effect'

c Is supplied in blue coloured cylinders

d Should only be administered to the patient by medical personnel

e The constituent gases can separate out at 5°C ambient temperature

chapter 1

PHYSICS

ANSWERS

1 Rotameters:

a **True** They are shaped like an inverted cone, so that the annular space around the bobbin is greater at the top of the tube than it is at the bottom.

b **True** Other forms of devices were used in the past, but modern bobbins with vanes cut into them rotate freely in the gas stream and are more accurate. There is very little friction between the light weight bobbins and the flow meter tube.

c **True** At low flows gas flow is laminar and at high flows it is turbulent. Calibration is necessary for each individual gas due to differences in density and viscosity.

d **False** At low flows, clearance around the bobbin is long and narrow, resembling a tube, and flow is usually laminar. At high flows the clearance is short and narrow, resembling an orifice, and flow becomes turbulent.

e **True** The flow from the emergency oxygen bypass and the from the top of the rotameter if the bobbin becomes stuck at the top have been found to be almost similar.

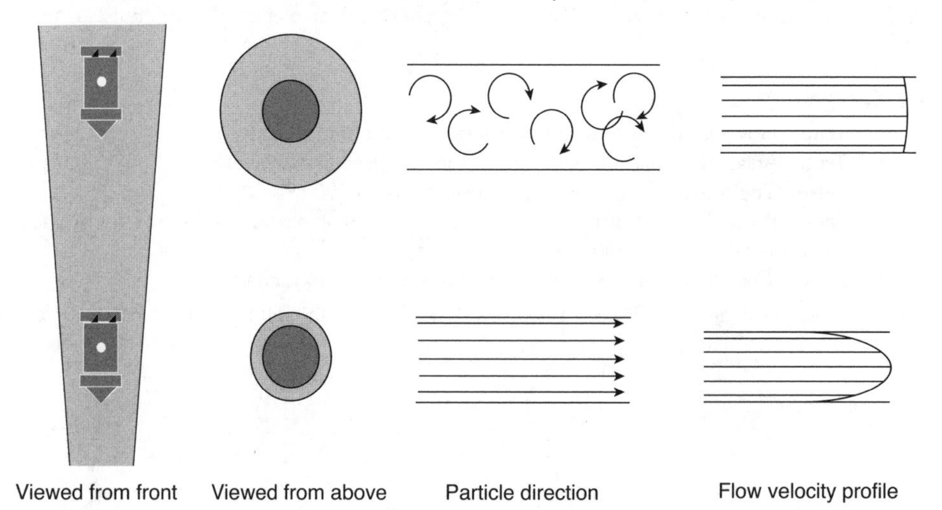

Figure 1.1 Flow in a rotameter.

Al-Shaikh B and Stacey S (2006) *Essentials of Anaesthetic Equipment*, 3rd edition. Edinburgh: Churchill Livingstone.
Davis P and Kenny G (2002) *Basic Physics and Measurement in Anaesthesia*, 5th edition. Boston, MA: Butterworth-Heinemann.
Kevin K and Spoors C (2009) *Training in Anaesthesia*. New York: Oxford University Press.

2 Regarding gases:

a **True** Since Entonox® is a gaseous mixture of nitrous oxide and oxygen, it is necessary to have a pressure of 137 bar in the cylinder to maintain the gaseous form.

b **False** Boyle's law states that the volume of a gas is inversely proportional to the pressure it is subjected to, the temperature remaining constant, i.e. $PV = K$ at constant temperature.

c **False** Flow is turbulent in the upper airways. The cross section of the lower airways is so much greater that the flow becomes laminar.

d **True** The critical velocity at which laminar flow changes to turbulent flow depends on the ratio of viscosity to density (n/p).

e **True** The most violent reaction occurs in a stoichiometric mixture. If the component concentrations change, the reaction will be less violent, or ignition may not occur at all.

Davis P and Kenny G (2002) *Basic Physics and Measurement in Anaesthesia*, 5th edition. Boston, MA: Butterworth-Heinemann.

3 Nitrogen:

a **True** The boiling point of nitrogen is –195.8°C and that of oxygen is –183°C.

b **False** Nitrogen is the slowest diffusing gas when compared with carbon dioxide, oxygen and nitrous oxide.

c **True** It is used in the storage of drugs such as thiopental (thiopentone).

d **True** As an inert gas, it can be safely used for this purpose.

e **True** Compressed air mixture used by divers can produce hallucinogenic effects that are time and depth dependent (nitrogen narcosis).

Davies N and Cashman J (1999) *Lee's Synopsis of Anaesthesia*. 13th edition. Oxford: Butterworth-Heinemann.

4 Oxygen:

a **True** However, this is not an economical method of manufacture.

b **True** Adiabatic expansion is the main principle used in manufacture.

c **False** The pressure inside an oxygen cylinder is 13 700 kPa.

d **True** It can diffuse in or out of the alveolus faster than nitrous oxide, nitrogen and air, but slower than carbon dioxide.

e **False** Oximetry measures the oxygen saturation not oxygen tension.

Davies N and Cashman J (1999) *Lee's Synopsis of Anaesthesia*. 13th edition. Oxford: Butterworth-Heinemann.

5 A wet spirometer can be used to directly measure:

a **True** The wet spirometer consists of a lightweight cylinder suspended over a breathing chamber with a water seal. Respiratory effort causes movement of the cylinder, which is recorded on a rotating drum by a pencil attached to the cylinder.

b **True** Inspiratory capacity is the maximum amount of air that can be breathed in at the end of a normal expiration. TV + IRV = inspiratory capacity, where TV is the tidal volume and IRV is the inspiratory reserve volume.

c **True** The wet spirometer can also be used to measure oxygen consumption. If the amount of oxygen in the breathing chamber at the start is known, oxygen consumption can be calculated.

d **False** The spirometer cannot measure the functional residual capacity (FRC) directly. It can be calculated by dilutional methods. Knowing the ERV + RV = FRC, the FRC can be derived using the nitrogen washout method (ERV, expiratory reserve volume; RV, residual volume).

e **True** Vital capacity (VC) = TV + IRV + ERV. TV, IRV, and ERV can all be directly measured with the wet spirometer.

Davis P and Kenny G (2002) *Basic Physics and Measurement in Anaesthesia*, 5th edition. Boston, MA: Butterworth-Heinemann.

6 Oxygen delivery systems:

a **False** Nasal cannulae can only deliver a maximum of 40% oxygen. The nasal mucosa dries up with high flows of oxygen, making nasal breathing painful. The patient resorts to mouth breathing causing dilution of inspired oxygen The optimum flow of oxygen is 2 l/min to prevent this problem.

b **True** High airflow oxygen entrainment (HAFOE) devices are the most efficient devices.

c **False** Since these masks deliver approximately 40 l/min flow, different masks delivering a fixed percentage of oxygen, each mask has its own fixed ratio for entrainment. For example a 24% mask may have a ratio of 19:1 (recommended oxygen flow 2 l/min) a 28% mask 9:1 (recommended oxygen flow 4 l/min) and a 35% mask 4:1 (recommended oxygen flow 8 l/min) to make up a total flow of 40 l/min. Only the 60% mask that delivers 30 l/min has an entrainment ratio of 1:1, i.e. 15 l of oxygen to 15 l of air. The flow delivery of 40 l/min is used for illustration purposes only, the actual flows from various masks and their air entrainment ratios may be different from those given above.

d **True** The flow rate should be equivalent to or greater than the patient's maximum inspiratory flow rate, approximately 30 l/min at rest.

e **True** Mapleson A (Magill's) is the only system to reliably deliver 100% oxygen.

Scurr C, Feldman S, and Soni N (1990) *Scientific Foundations of Anaesthesia*, 4th edition. Oxford: Butterworth-Heinemann.

7 Regarding humidification:

a **True** Room air contains only 16 mg/l of water. The alveolus contains 44 mg/l of water, therefore 28 mg of water must be added.

b **False** It is the temperature at which the partial pressure of water equals the saturated vapour. It gives an indication of relative humidity at that temperature.

c **True** A particle size of 5–10 μg is ideal for humidifying the terminal airways. Droplets of 20 μg would deposit in delivery tubing or upper airways.

d **True** Ultrasonic nebulizers used for humidification function at 2 MHz and produce 0–5 μg droplets, which can deposit in the alveoli and therefore can pose a risk of water overload and pulmonary oedema, especially in children.

e **True** The fall in pressure at points of constriction where flow velocity is high is known as the 'Bernoulli effect'. These changes allow entrainment of air at constriction points. This phenomenon is used in the apparatus using the Venturi principle such as oxygen masks and nebulizers.

Davis P and Kenny G (2002) *Basic Physics and Measurement in Anaesthesia*, 5th edition. Boston, MA: Butterworth-Heinemann.

8 Cardiac output can be measured by:

a **True** Indocyanine green is injected into a central vein. Blood is sampled from an arterial cannula and change in dye concentration over time is measured. The area under the concentration/time curve corresponds to the cardiac output. This technique is limited by dye accumulation preventing rapid repeat measurements.

b **True** Using a pulmonary artery catheter, cold saline is injected into the right atrium, the change in temperature being measured by the catheter thermistor within the pulmonary artery. A computer calculates the cardiac output using the Stewart–Hamilton equation. Cardiac output is inversely proportional to the area under the temperature/time curve.

c **True** A low-amplitude, high-frequency alternating current is produced between neck and chest electrodes. The electrical impedance is measured and represents the thoracic impedance. Changes in pulsatile blood flow produce a change in impedance, and from this stroke volume is estimated. Cardiac output can then be calculated.

d **False** It is used for measuring lung volumes and pressures.

e **True** This technique is difficult to perform and rarely used. It involves detection of motion resulting from movement of blood within the body occurring with each heart beat.

Pinnock C, Lin T, and Smith T (2002) *Fundamentals of Anaesthesia*, 2nd edition. New York: Cambridge University Press.

9 Oxygen analysis can be performed using the following apparatus:

a **True** It is measured by the polarographic method. The measurement is accurate to within 2 mmHg.

b **True** Oxygen analysis can be performed by the manometric or volumetric method. This method is not used clinically.

c **False** The Daniel cell is an early version of the battery.

d **True** By amplifying the released electrons from the oxygen and fuel reaction the oxygen concentration can be estimated. The fuel cell degrades over time, like an ordinary battery.

e **False** The Weston cell is a wet cell that was used for calibration of voltmeters in the past.

Davis P and Kenny G (2002) *Basic Physics and Measurement in Anaesthesia*, 5th edition. Boston, MA: Butterworth-Heinemann.

10 The Vitalograph:

a **True** This a lightweight version of the wet spirometer. The inertia of the bell and pulleys of the wet spirometer can produce inaccuracies, which have been eliminated in this device.
b **True** It has a chart that depicts the waveform with necessary corrections.
c **True** The device measures FEV_1 and many other parameters, and displays the measurements on a chart.
d **True** PEFR can be obtained using the Vitalograph; the predicted value and percentage is also displayed.
e **True** Since this is a mathematical derivation, FEV_1 would suffice to calculate the MVV.

Davis P and Kenny G (2002) *Basic Physics and Measurement in Anaesthesia*, 5th edition. Boston, MA: Butterworth-Heinemann.

11 Infrared analysers can be used for the estimation of:

a **True** This method is employed by the capnograph in measuring carbon dioxide
b **True** Each diatomic gas absorbs infrared radiation at a characteristic wavelength. Choosing infrared radiation with a particular wavelength makes it possible to measure individual gases.
c **True** Infrared radiation passes through the sample chamber onto a photodetector. The more infrared radiation that is absorbed, the less is detected by the photodetector. This signal is processed electronically to indicate the concentration of gas in the chamber.
d **True** Halothane concentration used to be measured by the ultraviolet absorption method.
e **False** Infrared radiation in the range of 1–15 μm is absorbed by all gases with more than two different atoms. Oxygen, not possessing dissimilar atoms, does not absorb infrared radiation and cannot be measured by this method.

Davis P and Kenny G (2002) *Basic Physics and Measurement in Anaesthesia*, 5th edition. Boston, MA: Butterworth-Heinemann.

12 PEEP:

a **True** The pressure during expiration stays at the set pressure above zero, thus preventing collapse of the alveoli.
b **True** It is positive end-expiratory pressure.
c **True** A PEEP valve provides almost constant expiratory resistance over a wide range of flow rates.
d **True** Over 10 cmH_2O pressure, the chances of barotrauma, and also of a reduction in cardiac output, are higher.
e **True** If the cardiac output has been affected adversely by reduced venous return, tissue oxygenation may not be efficient.

Al-Shaikh B and Stacey S (2006) *Essentials of Anaesthetic Equipment*, 3rd edition. Edinburgh: Churchill Livingstone.

13 The following are examples of pressure release devices:

a **False** A Bourdon gauge measures pressure; increasing gas pressure leads to uncoiling of a tube and movement of a pointer over a dial.
b **False** Aneroid gauge is another name for the Bourdon gauge, from the Greek *a-neros* ('without liquid').
c **True** It has been used routinely with an Ambu bag.
d **True** This was the most commonly used expiratory valve in the past with most of the breathing circuits, Mapleson A to D.
e **True** It is an expiratory valve used in the USA.

Al-Shaikh B and Stacey S (2006) *Essentials of Anaesthetic Equipment*, 3rd edition. Edinburgh: Churchill Livingstone.

14 Soda lime:

a **False** The components are: calcium hydroxide 94%; sodium hydroxide 5%; potassium hydroxide 1%; and silica 0.2%.
b **False** The particles should be 4–8 mesh in size. The smaller the size, the greater the possibility of inhaling dust particles from the canister.
c **True** Mapleson C is a Waters circuit used for resuscitation and in recovery. It is possible to add a soda lime canister to it to prevent rebreathing of carbon dioxide.
d **True** Such a possibility has been documented, particularly after a period of disuse where drying out has occurred.
e **True** Historically, with the use of trichloroethylene, cranial nerve V and VII palsies were reported at a temperature of 60°C. Modern soda lime formulations do not allow the temperature to rise above 40°C. Trichloroethylene was the first agent to be licensed for midwives to administer for analgesia in labour.

Aitkenhead A and Smith G (2008) *Textbook of Anaesthesia*, 5th edition. Edinburgh: Churchill Livingstone.

15 A transducer:

a **False** It is a device that converts one form of energy to another.
b **True** As in cardiac catheterization and in pulmonary artery catheters.
c **True** The arterial pulsations are transmitted along the saline column on to the transducer, which forms one limb of the Wheatstone bridge.
d **True** A light beam is transmitted along a medium, e.g. blood, and the intensity of the reflected beam is detected. This principle has been used in cardiac catheter studies.
e **True** Since a continuous reading of blood pressure is a dynamic process it can lead to distortion of the wave form. The higher harmonics of an arterial pressure wave form lie in the range of 20 cycles per second. Hence a transducer system with a resonant frequency of 30 cycles per second will respond satisfactorily to arterial pressure changes.

Davis P and Kenny G (2002) *Basic Physics and Measurement in Anaesthesia*, 5th edition. Boston, MA: Butterworth-Heinemann.

16 Vaporizers:

a **True** The draw-over principle was used by vaporizers in the past. Gas is pushed through the vaporizer under pressure, at a steady rate. Only a small fraction of it is diverted to the vaporizing chamber, which collects the vapour and then rejoins the main stream. This way a steady flow of vapour is delivered at the patient end, without appreciable cooling of the volatile agent within the vaporizer.

b **True** Temperature changes from loss of latent heat of vaporization are compensated by making the vaporizer from a material with a high specific heat capacity and high thermal conductivity, e.g. copper, and having a temperature sensitive splitting valve, e.g. bimetallic strip, which allows more gas into the vaporizing chamber as temperature falls thus maintaining constant output.

c **False** Wicks in the vaporizing chamber are usually made of copper, which is the most efficient for providing heat exchange.

d **True** Since the product of volume × density remains the same, output from the vaporizer will be accurate.

e **False** Efficient vaporizers have a very high resistance to respiration and there is a risk of a constantly increasing agent concentration and they should therefore never be used inside a circle. An inefficient vaporizer, e.g. Goldman, enables easy breathing, and the resultant cooling of the agent also reduces the vapour pressure, thus acting as a safety device.

Al-Shaikh B and Stacey S (2006) *Essentials of Anaesthetic Equipment*, 3rd edition. Edinburgh: Churchill Livingstone.

Davis P and Kenny G (2002) *Basic Physics and Measurement in Anaesthesia*, 5th edition. Boston, MA: Butterworth-Heinemann.

17 During anaesthesia under hyperbaric conditions:

a **False** In normal conditions nitrous oxide does not promote combustion but under hyperbaric conditions it does and therefore should be avoided.

b **False** They are not affected by pressure changes.

c **True** The density of gases is increased under hyperbaric conditions so the flow meters will read higher than the actual flow through them.

d **True** The air within the endotracheal tube cuff can expand suddenly during decompression and cause rupture of the trachea. Unless constant cuff pressure monitoring is used the cuff should be filled with water or saline.

e **False** For similar reasons as above, glass bottles of infusions or medications should be avoided.

Aitkenhead A and Smith G (2008) *Textbook of Anaesthesia*, 5th edition. Edinburgh: Churchill Livingstone.

18 The following may be used for sterilization of equipment:

a **True** Formaldehyde has been used until recently for sterilizing anaesthetic machines.

b **False** Infrared has not been used for this purpose.

c **True** Many of the bulky disposable items such as oxygenators used in cardiopulmonary bypass circuits are sterilized with gamma radiation. It is more expensive than other methods.

d **False** Ethanol is ethyl alcohol and is not used in sterilizing equipment.

e **False** It is a coolant used in industry. During the synthesis of glycol, ethylene oxide is produced and is a very useful sterilizing agent. Ethylene oxide, however, is used for sterilizing many products, including needles, cannulae and endotracheal tubes.

Al-Shaikh B and Stacey S (2006) *Essentials of Anaesthetic Equipment*, 3rd edition. Edinburgh: Churchill Livingstone.

19 The hot air oven is not as efficient as an autoclave because:

a **True** Dry heat at 150°C must be applied for 30 minutes to sterilize equipment. An autoclave uses moist heat (steam under pressure) and requires less heat for shorter periods of time: at 134°C and a pressure of 3 atm, sterility is achieved in just three minutes.

b **True** This illustrates how inefficient dry heat is compared to the autoclaving process. However, not all materials are suitable for autoclaving, for example plastic, as it would melt. Therefore other methods are still required.

c **True** Using dry heat means that a longer time is required for the heat to transfer to the microorganism. It is particularly important that any physical dirt is removed to aid this process.

d **False** Dry heat kills by oxidation whereas moist heat kills by coagulation of protein.

e **True** Wet heat kills microorganism faster than dry heat. To remove prion proteins much longer periods of exposure are required as prions are particularly resistant.

Macintosh R, Mushin WW, and Epstein HG (1987) *Physics for the Anaesthetist*. Oxford: Blackwell Scientific.

Pinnock C, Lin T, and Smith T (2002) *Fundamentals of Anaesthesia*, 2nd edition. New York: Cambridge University Press.

20 Concerning the gas laws:

a **False** Boyle's law describes the relationship between volume and pressure at constant temperature.

b **True** Thus, the total pressure of a mixture of gases equals the sum of pressures of individual gases.

c **False** Henry's law states that at a given temperature the amount of gas dissolved in a liquid is proportional to the partial pressure of the gas in equilibrium with the liquid. Henry's law explains how nitrogen under pressure enters the tissues of a diver as they descend. If they then ascend too rapidly the nitrogen comes out of the tissues as bubbles leading to the symptoms of decompression sickness (the bends).

d **True** Gay Lussac's law describes the relationship between pressure and temperature of a gas at constant volume. If a constant volume of gas is heated, the pressure will increase.

e **False** Charles' law states that at constant pressure the volume of a gas is proportional to its absolute temperature.

Davis P and Kenny G (2002) *Basic Physics and Measurement in Anaesthesia*, 5th edition. Boston, MA: Butterworth-Heinemann.

21 The following gases are lighter than air:

a **False** Nitrous oxide is heavier than air.

b **False** Cyclopropane is heavier than air.

c **False** Carbon dioxide is heavier than air.

d **False** Diethyl ether is heavier than air.

e **True** Apart from ethylene oxide, other common gases that are lighter than air are ammonia, nitrogen, hydrogen, and helium.

Davies N and Cashman J (1999) *Lee's Synopsis of Anaesthesia*. 13th edition. Oxford: Butterworth-Heinemann.

22 Concerning flow of a gas or liquid through a tube:

a **True** As the viscosity increases, the resistance to flow increases. Flow resistance, *R*, is proportional to the length of the tube and the viscosity of the fluid, and inversely related to the fourth power of the radius.

b **False** Flow rate is proportional to the pressure across the tube and to the fourth power of radius. Laminar flow is not affected by density.

c **False** Resistance is inversely proportional to the fourth power and not the square of the radius.

d **True** When the critical velocity is reached the flow turns from laminar to turbulent and energy is lost as friction between the layers of fluid.

e **True** Turbulent flow is directly proportional to the square root of the pressure across the tube.

Davis P and Kenny G (2002) *Basic Physics and Measurement in Anaesthesia*, 5th edition. Boston, MA: Butterworth-Heinemann.

23 In statistical terms:

a **True** The variable may be on a continuous scale, e.g. weight, or may be discrete, e.g. blood group.

b **True** When describing normally distributed data, the mean indicates central tendency.

c **False** Degrees of freedom, *N*, is the number of observations available for comparison and is therefore equal to $n - 1$.

d **True** In a normally distributed sample, the mode and median also equal the mean, this can be a useful test of whether the distribution is in fact normal.

e **False** Variance (σ^2) is a measure of variation about the mean. It is calculated by the equation:

$$\text{Variance } (\sigma^2) = \frac{\sum (\text{measured value} - \text{mean})^2}{(n - 1)}$$

Where $\sum$ = sum and n – 1 equals the degrees of freedom.

Pinnock C, Lin T, and Smith T (2002) *Fundamentals of Anaesthesia*, 2nd edition. New York: Cambridge University Press.

24 Statistical tests of significance include:

a **True** Used for comparing data from two normally distributed samples. Calculates 't':

$$t = \frac{\text{Difference between the means}}{\text{Standard error of the difference}}$$

b **True** Similar to the Mann–Whitney U-test, this is used for non-normally distributed data. Each variable is assigned a ranking score and the calculation is performed with these scores rather than the value to eliminate the effect of skewed data. Not to be confused with Wilcoxon's signed rank test, which is used to compare two non-normally distributed samples with paired data.

c **True** Sequential analysis involves analysing study data as it is collected. Clinical trials have been stopped early when sequential analysis has shown a clear benefit of a drug, or clear mortality difference between groups.

d **True** The chi-squared test is used for qualitative data, with Fisher's exact test if >20% of the expected frequencies are <5.

e **True** A dependent variable can be plotted against an independent variable which is changed and the relationship between them, if any, can be determined. This can be open to misinterpretation and confounding factors.

Pinnock C, Lin T, and Smith T (2002) *Fundamentals of Anaesthesia*, 2nd edition. New York: Cambridge University Press.

25 The apparatus listed have the following uses:

a **False** The oximeter measures the saturation and not tension.

b **False** It measures flow. It can be used in conjunction with other devices to determine airway resistance.

c **False** It is used for measuring the cardiac output.

d **True** It is used for determination of many inorganic ions.

e **False** A gas with high thermal conductivity conducts heat more readily than one with a low conductivity. Katharometers study the degree of cooling of a heated wire when a particular gas is passed over it and calculate the concentration of the gas.

Davis P and Kenny G (2002) *Basic Physics and Measurement in Anaesthesia*, 5th edition. Boston, MA: Butterworth-Heinemann.

26 Doppler-shift instruments are used for:

a **True** A Doppler device may be used to measure blood flow. Colour Doppler uses colour superimposed on the greyscale image with flow away from the probe represented as red and towards the probe as blue. Different colours may also be used to indicate the velocity of the blood flow.

b **True** The movement of the arterial wall under a pressure cuff can be detected by Doppler. Systolic and diastolic blood pressure is determined by the amplitude of Doppler shifts. This method is particularly sensitive to movement artefact.

c **True** Doppler probes have been placed over the internal jugular vein during procedures with high risk of gas embolism, for example neurosurgery in a seated patient. However, this method has a high rate of false positives from clinically insignificant volumes of air and is less used now.

d **True** Doppler devices can be used to continuously monitor movement of the chest and can therefore be employed as apnoea monitors, for example in paediatric intensive care units.

e **True** Stroke volume is measured by directing the beam at the arch of aorta, and the velocity signal is multiplied by the cross-sectional area of the aorta and then integrated with respect to time during the ejection phase of the cycle. Cardiac output can then be obtained by multiplying this value by the heart rate per minute.

Davis P and Kenny G (2002) *Basic Physics and Measurement in Anaesthesia*, 5th edition. Boston, MA: Butterworth-Heinemann.

27 Regarding radiation:

a **True** The atomic number is also referred to as the proton number and is the number of protons in the nucleus of the atom.

b **False** Isotopes are atoms with the same number of protons and electrons but extra neutrons. Thus their atomic number remains the same but the atomic mass number (protons plus neutrons) increases.

c **False** Biological half-life refers to the disappearance of a substance from a particular organ or tissue and may depend on metabolism and blood flow, whereas the physical half-life is rate of decay of an isotope and cannot be altered by any physical process.

d **True** Gamma radiation is used in the sterilization of disposable anaesthetic equipment. However it is more expensive and potentially hazardous than other methods.

e **True** A Geiger counter is a standard device used to detect free radiation.

Davis P and Kenny G (2002) *Basic Physics and Measurement in Anaesthesia*, 5th edition. Boston, MA: Butterworth-Heinemann.

28 For ventilating a patient with high airway resistance:

a **False** A constant pressure ventilator would not be able to generate any extra pressure to overcome any change in the airway resistance.

b **True** By increasing the tidal volume, the volume lost due to compression could be compensated for, but this has to be done with simultaneously slowing of the respiratory rate.

c **False** There is no advantage in increasing the inspiratory flow rate.

d **False** Slowing the respiratory rate gives more time to the gases to equilibrate.

e **False** NEEP will cause airways to collapse before complete emptying of the lungs has occurred and would cause air trapping with disastrous consequences, such as pneumothorax.

Aitkenhead A and Smith G. (2008) *Textbook of Anaesthesia*, 5th edition. Edinburgh: Churchill Livingstone.

29 Anaesthetic breathing circuits:

a **True** Mapleson D, also known as the Bain circuit, is the most efficient for invasive positive pressure ventilation (IPPV).

b **True** The fresh gas flow is distal to the expiratory valve, and fresh gas flow in excess of twice the minute ventilation is required for both spontaneous and controlled ventilation. This system is not in use in current practice.

c **False** Lack circuit is the co-axial version of Mapleson A or Magill's circuit, which is the most efficient for spontaneous ventilation. A flow rate to match the alveolar ventilation is adequate.

d **False** Jackson Rees modified the Mapleson E circuit, producing the Mapleson F circuit, which is suitable for IPPV and spontaneous ventilation in children <20 kg.

e **True** A resistance greater than given would make spontaneous ventilation more strenuous.

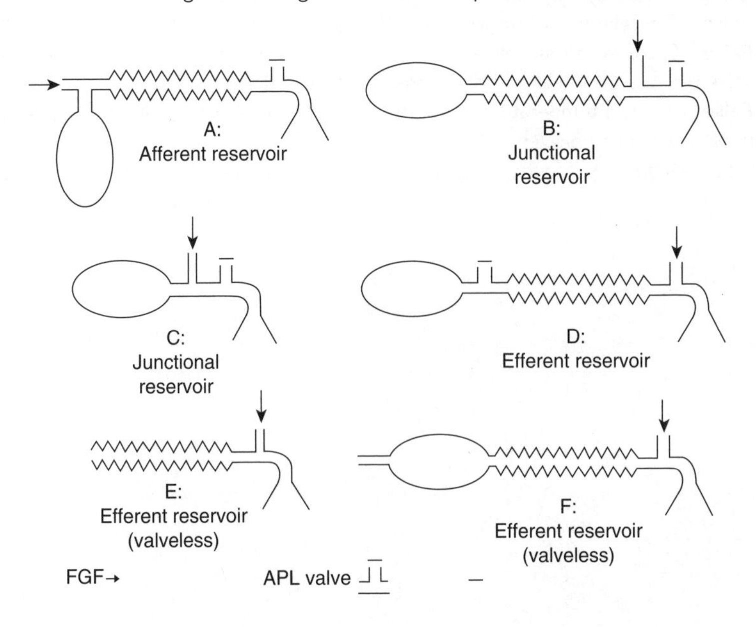

Figure 1.2 Mapleson classification.
Reproduced with kind permission from Kevin K and Spoors C (2009) *Training in Anaesthesia*. New York: Oxford University Press.

Table 1.4 Anaesthetic breathing systems

	A	B	C	D	E and F	Circle
Spontaneous breathing	In theory, alveolar minute volume; in practice, minute volume	2–3 × minute volume	2–3 × minute volume	2–3 × minute volume	2–3 × minute volume	*In theory,* only the patient's oxygen consumption (once primed with fresh gas and volatile)
Intermittent positive pressure ventilation	2–3 × minute volume	2–3 × minute volume	2–3 × minute volume	70–100 ml/kg/min	200–300 ml/kg/min	

IPPV, invasive positive pressure ventilation; FGF, fresh gas flow.

Aitkenhead A and Smith G (2008) *Textbook of Anaesthesia*, 5th edition. Edinburgh: Churchill Livingstone.
Kevin K and Spoors C (2009) *Training in Anaesthesia*. New York: Oxford University Press.

30 Entonox®:

a **True** This was the only way of making sure that both nitrous oxide and oxygen remain in a gaseous form.
b **True** Poynting was the engineer with BOC who came up with this solution; hence it is known as the 'Poynting effect'.
c **False** The cylinder is blue with white and blue quarters on the shoulder.
d **False** Entonox® should always be self-administered by the patient. Using a demand valve reduces the likelihood of unconsciousness in the patient.
e **False** Below a temperature of –5.5°C, nitrous oxide will laminate out of a mixture of nitrous oxide and oxygen.

Aitkenhead A and Smith G (2008) *Textbook of Anaesthesia*, 5th edition. Edinburgh: Churchill Livingstone.

chapter 1 PHYSIOLOGY

QUESTIONS

1 Functional residual capacity (FRC):

a Is normally around 1.5 litres in a 70 kg adult male
b Is the amount of gas present in the lung after maximal expiration
c Is affected by age
d Decreases under general anaesthesia
e Is less affected by neuraxial block than general anaesthesia

2 Concerning vital capacity:

a It is the maximum volume of air that can be expired at the end of a normal expiration
b The volume is approximately 3.5 litres
c It is decreased in old age
d It is decreased by 17% in the lithotomy position
e A vital capacity breath uses the third to seventh intercostal muscles in addition to the diaphragm and abdominal muscles

3 Compliance of the lungs:

a Is equal to the change in volume per unit increase in intrathoracic pressure
b Is equal to the thoracic compliance
c Is less in infants than in young adults
d Is reduced in emphysema
e Is approximately 200 ml/cmH_2O

4 The following volumes constitute the vital capacity:

a Tidal volume
b Inspiratory reserve volume
c Functional residual capacity (FRC)
d Residual volume
e Expiratory reserve volume

5 The following are normal values in a healthy adult male:

a FEV_1 – 3.9 litres
b FRC – 4 litres
c IRV – 2 litres
d RV – 2.5 litres
e Maximal voluntary ventilation (MVV) or maximal breathing capacity (MBC) – 125–170 l/min

6 Closing volume:

- a Is the volume at which all the airways are closed
- b Can be measured using radioactive xenon
- c Is inversely proportional to age
- d Increases under general anaesthesia
- e Is directly affected by the supine position

7 Carbon dioxide:

- a Is produced at a rate of 250 ml/min at rest
- b Is 20 times more soluble than oxygen
- c Is carried mostly as bicarbonate in the plasma
- d Is carried to a smaller extent (one-fifth) as a carbamino compound by haemoglobin
- e Has a tension of 6.0 kPa in venous blood

8 The following are associated with various forms of hypoxia:

- a Arterial oxygen tension is decreased, oxygen saturation is normal in 'anaemic hypoxia'
- b Arterial oxygen saturation is decreased, oxygen tension is normal in 'stagnant hypoxia'
- c Venous oxygen content is decreased in 'hypoxic hypoxia'
- d Arterio-venous oxygen difference is increased in 'diffusion hypoxia'
- e Cyanosis is a significant feature in 'histotoxic hypoxia'

9 A raised PCO_2 occurs in:

- a Acute air embolism
- b Chronic bronchitis
- c Renal failure
- d Persistent vomiting
- e Diabetic ketoacidosis

10 Anaemia:

- a Is a haemoglobin level below 13 g/dl in the male
- b May be caused by chronic blood loss
- c May be secondary to rheumatoid arthritis
- d May occur with hypothyroidism
- e Is a recognized feature of chronic renal impairment

11 Cyanosis:

- a Is a feature of hypercarbia
- b Is seen in iron deficiency anaemia
- c Is seen when there is 2 g/100 ml of reduced haemoglobin
- d Is frequently seen in polycythaemia rubra vera
- e Is an early feature of cyanide poisoning

12 Regarding the speed of diffusion of air, oxygen, carbon dioxide, nitrogen, and nitrous oxide through the alveolus:

a Oxygen diffuses the fastest
b Carbon dioxide diffuses slower than oxygen
c Nitrous oxide diffuses slower than oxygen and carbon dioxide
d Nitrogen diffuses slower than oxygen, carbon dioxide, and nitrous oxide
e Air diffuses the slowest of all the gases

13 Increasing the intrathoracic pressure to 40 cmH_2O in a normal person produce the following changes initially:

a Decrease in blood pressure
b Decrease in peripheral vascular resistance
c Increase in stroke volume
d Increase in heart rate
e Increase in frequency of baroreceptor discharge

14 Hyperventilation:

a Will decrease plasma pH
b Will decrease ionized calcium levels
c Will cause metabolic alkalosis
d Will increase the standard bicarbonate
e Can cause hypotension

15 At high altitude:

a Oxygen tension is reduced
b Oxygen percentage is reduced
c The viscosity of air is reduced
d Hyperventilation must occur to compensate for hypoxic hypoxia
e Pulmonary arterial pressure increases

16 Alveolar–arterial oxygen difference:

a Is an important indicator of venous admixture
b Is 0.5–1 kPa normally
c Increases under general anaesthesia
d Is increased in hypovolaemia
e Is increased by low inspired oxygen concentration

17 Cardiac index

a Is cardiac output × body weight
b Is cardiac output × total peripheral resistance
c Is left ventricular pressure minus left atrial pressure
d Is greater in males than females
e Is 3.2 l/m^2 surface area

18 With respect to the lungs:

a Compliance is greater when the lungs are enclosed in the thorax than when exposed to the atmosphere
b Pulmonary blood flow equals alveolar ventilation at rest
c The diffusion capacity of the lungs for oxygen is normally 50 ml/min/mmHg at rest
d Pulmonary blood volume increases by approximately 400 ml in the supine position
e Inactivation of bradykinin, serotonin, and prostaglandin occurs in the lungs

19 Basal metabolic rate (BMR):

a Is 3500 kcal per day
b Is increased in the female
c Is increased in tropical climates
d Is decreased during sleep
e Is decreased in the elderly

20 Factors leading to increased insulin secretion include:

a Noradrenaline (norepinephrine)
b Glucagon
c Phenytoin
d Beta blockers
e Sulphonylureas

21 Features of restrictive lung disorders include:

a A reduction in the FEV_1:FVC ratio
b Reduced peak expiratory flow rate (PEFR)
c Reduced transfer factor to carbon monoxide
d Normal residual volume
e Normal total lung capacity

22 Surfactant:

a Decreases the surface tension of the liquid lining the air spaces of the lung
b Increases the lung compliance
c Increases the amount of fluid within the alveoli
d Allows expansion of alveoli at a pressure of 0.8–1 kPa
e Is absent at 35 weeks' gestation

23 Airway resistance:

a Can be measured using a body plethysmograph
b Can be measured with a peak flow meter
c Can be measured with a pneumotachograph
d Is greater during inspiration than expiration during an asthma attack
e Is greater in the terminal bronchioles than the upper airways

24 Compensatory measures in response to metabolic acidosis include:

a Decreased $PaCO_2$
b Increased bicarbonate excretion
c Increased sodium excretion
d Decreased ammonia excretion
e Increased potassium excretion

25 Excessive secretion of mineralocorticoids:

a Increase serum potassium levels
b Increase circulating blood volume
c Increase urinary sodium excretion
d Is associated with metabolic alkalosis
e Is associated with hyperglycaemia

26 Antidiuretic hormone (ADH):

a Is produced by the posterior pituitary gland
b Increases reabsorption of water in the proximal convoluted tubule
c Increases permeability of the distal convoluted tubule to water
d Increases permeability of the collecting duct to water
e Increases the osmolality of urine

27 Cardiac output:

a Is stroke volume × heart rate
b Is increased by late pregnancy
c Decreases during sleep
d Is decreased up to 30% by standing from the supine position
e Is decreased by adrenaline (epinephrine)

28 Anatomical dead space:

a Can be correlated to body weight
b Is greater while standing upright
c Is increased when the neck is extended and the jaw protruded
d Is increased by administration of atropine
e Varies directly with the tidal volume (about one-third of tidal volume)

29 Physiological dead space:

a Is measured using the Bohr equation
b Is affected by the $PaCO_2$
c Is affected by the tidal volume
d Is increased by low cardiac output
e Can be assumed to be the same as the anatomical dead space in normal individuals

30 Left atrial pressure:

a Is around 0–2 mmHg
b Is usually reflected by the pulmonary capillary wedge pressure (PCWP)
c May produce left heart failure at pressures greater than 15 mmHg
d Is a better guide to fluid balance in heart failure
e Causes pulmonary oedema when it exceeds 30 mmHg

chapter 1 PHYSIOLOGY

ANSWERS

1 Functional residual capacity (FRC):

a **False** It is usually around 2.2 litres in men and 1.8 litres in women.

b **False** FRC is the volume of gas left in the lungs after a normal expiration (FRC = ERV + RV, where ERV is the expiratory reserve volume and RV is the residual volume).

c **True** FRC decreases with age.

d **True** FRC is decreased under general anaesthesia (up to 20%) under spontaneous and even with controlled ventilation. The mechanism is not clear but is thought to involve decrease in muscular tone.

e **True** FRC is less affected by neuraxial blocks than general anaesthesia. Factors that decrease FRC include: age, posture, anaesthesia, surgery, pulmonary fibrosis, pulmonary oedema, obesity, abdominal swelling, thoracic wall distortion, and reduced muscle tone.

Factors that increase FRC include: positive end-expiratory pressure (PEEP)/continuous positive airway pressure (CPAP), increased airway resistance, e.g. in asthma, and exercise, which increases inspiratory muscular tone.

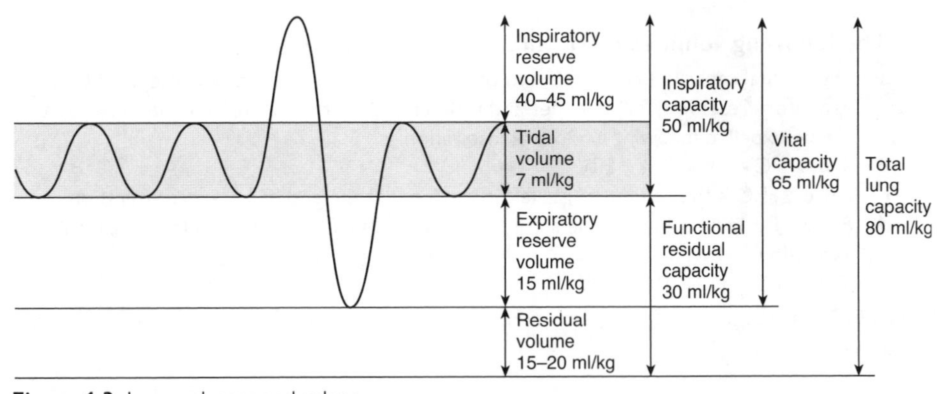

Figure 1.3 Lung volumes and values.

Aitkenhead A and Smith G (2008) *Textbook of Anaesthesia*, 5th edition. Edinburgh: Churchill Livingstone.

Barrett K, Barman S, Boitano S, and Brooks HL (2009) *Ganong's Review of Medical Physiology*, 23rd edition. USA: McGraw-Hill.

Kevin K and Spoors C (2009) *Training in Anaesthesia*. New York: Oxford University Press

Yentis S, Hirsh N, and Smith G (2003) *Anaesthesia and Intensive Care A to Z*, 3rd edition. London: Butterworth-Heinemann.

2 Concerning vital capacity:

a **False** It is the volume that can be expelled completely after a maximal inspiration.
b **False** It is usually around 4500 ml.
c **True** It can decrease by approximately 1 litre by the age of 70 years.
d **True** The abdominal contents push upwards, splinting the diaphragm and decreasing the vital capacity.
e **False** The fourth to ninth intercostal muscles are involved in increasing the anteroposterior and transverse diameters of the thorax, producing the bucket handle action of the ribs.

Pocock G and Richards C (2004) *Human Physiology: The basis of medicine*, 3rd edition. Oxford: Oxford University Press.

3 Compliance of the lungs:

a **False** Compliance is change in lung volume per unit change in pressure. This is transpulmonary pressure not intrathoracic pressure.
b **True** Thoracic compliance is the sum of lung compliance and chest wall compliance. Both are given a value of 200 ml/cmH_2O.
c **True** The lung compliance in the neonate is 5 ml/cmH_2O.
d **False** Lung compliance is increased, the lungs lose their elasticity and the walls between the alveoli break down, and the alveoli are replaced by large air sacs. The opposing recoil of the lung declines, and the chest becomes enlarged and barrel shaped. So the overall thoracic compliance decreases.
e **True** Lung compliance is 200 ml/cmH_2O or 2 l/kPa.

Barrett K, Barman S, Boitano S, and Brooks HL (2009) *Ganong's Review of Medical Physiology*, 23rd edition. USA: McGraw-Hill.

4 The following volumes constitute the vital capacity:

a **True** Vital capacity (VC) is the sum of tidal volume (TV), inspiratory reserve (IRV) and expiratory reserve (ERV) volumes and is described as the maximal volume of gas that can be expelled following a maximal inspiration.
b **True** VC = TV + IRV + ERV.
c **False** FRC is the volume of gas left in the lungs at the end of a normal expiration.
d **False** Residual volume is the amount of gas that is left in the lungs after a maximal expiration.
e **True** VC = TV + IRV + ERV.

Barrett K, Barman S, Boitano S, and Brooks HL (2009) *Ganong's Review of Medical Physiology*, 23rd edition. USA: McGraw-Hill.

5 The following are normal values in a healthy adult male:

a **False** The normal FEV_1 is between around 3 litres and 3.6 litres, which is 70–80% of the vital capacity (4.5 litres approximately).

b **False** FRC is approximately 2.2 litres in men and 1.8 litres in women.

c **False** IRV is around 3.8 litres in men and 2.5 litres in women.

d **False** RV is about 1.2 litres in men and about the same in women.

e **True** The MVV or MBC per minute is the amount of air that a person can breathe in and out rapidly. It gives an assessment regarding the voluntary effort that the person can generate. However, since this is a very strenuous test a mathematical approximation is used. MVV/MBC is approximately $FEV_1 \times 35$ (the number of breaths that can be generated in a minute) = MVV in l/min.

Pinnock C, Lin T, and Smith T (2002) *Fundamentals of Anaesthesia*, 2nd edition. New York: Cambridge University Press.
Yentis S, Hirsh N, and Smith G (2003) *Anaesthesia and Intensive Care A to Z*, 3rd edition. London: Butterworth-Heinemann.

6 Closing volume:

a **False** Closing volume is the volume at which dependent airways begin to close during expiration. Closing capacity is the closing volume plus residual volume.

b **True** A single breath washout technique with either helium or xenon may be used. The concentration of helium or xenon is measured during a slow expiration. A sharp rise in concentration of the gas is seen at the closing volume.

c **False** The closing volume increases with age and may encroach on the FRC. By the age of 45, closing volume encroaches on the FRC when supine, and by the age of 65, closing volume encroaches on the FRC when upright.

d **True** Closing volume is increased and FRC is decreased under anaesthesia This can lead to areas of lung collapse during normal expiration.

e **False** Closing volume is not affected by position.

Barrett K, Barman S, Boitano S, and Brooks HL (2009) *Ganong's Review of Medical Physiology*, 23rd edition. USA: McGraw-Hill.

7 Carbon dioxide:

a **False** Normal production of carbon dioxide is 200 ml/min but depends on the energy source used.

b **True** Carbon dioxide is 20 times more soluble than oxygen so is partly carried in dissolved form (around 8% is carried in solution in the blood).

c **True** Most of the carbon dioxide approximately 70%, is carried in the plasma as bicarbonate.

d **True** 22% is carried as carbamino compounds formed by reactions of carbon dioxide with amino groups of proteins. Haemoglobin provides most of the proteins. Deoxyhaemoglobin is able to bind more carbon dioxide than oxyhaemoglobin. This is principle behind the Haldane effect.

e **True** Arterial blood has a PCO_2 of 5.3 kPa. Addition of carbon dioxide by the tissues raises the PCO_2 in venous blood by 0.7 kPa to 6 kPa.

Pinnock C, Lin T, and Smith T (2002) *Fundamentals of Anaesthesia*, 2nd edition. New York: Cambridge University Press.

8 The following are associated with various forms of hypoxia:

a **False** Oxygen tension and the saturation may be normal but the haemoglobin available is decreased.

b **False** There is normal arterial PO_2 and haemoglobin but reduced tissue blood flow due to interrupted blood flow or low cardiac output.

c **True** Since there is lowering of arterial oxygen content there is a similar fall in venous content.

d **True** This is a similar picture to hypoxic hypoxia and hence will exhibit a greater arterio-venous oxygen difference.

e **False** In histotoxic hypoxia, the tissues are unable extract the oxygen from the haemoglobin and patients usually exhibit a healthy colour, e.g. cherry red in carbon monoxide poisoning and in cyanide poisoning. A bedside diagnosis of cyanide poisoning (as may occur after sodium nitroprusside infusion) is achieved by inspection of a drop of blood from a finger prick, which appears arterial in colour.

Barrett K, Barman S, Boitano S, and Brooks HL (2009) *Ganong's Review of Medical Physiology*, 23rd edition. USA: McGraw-Hill.

9 A raised PCO_2 occurs in:

a **False** The cardinal sign of air embolism is a sudden and large fall in end tidal carbon dioxide which would be similarly reflected in the arterial tension acutely as the resulting hypoxaemia leads to hyperventilation and hypocapnia.

b **True** Inefficient gas exchange would result in an elevation in some cases.

c **False** Decreased ability of the kidneys to efficiently excrete hydrogen ions leads to metabolic acidosis and corresponding decrease in carbon dioxide as a compensatory mechanism.

d **True** Persistent vomiting resulting in metabolic alkalosis may be compensated by a degree of respiratory acidosis.

e **False** Diabetic ketoacidosis causes the patient to hyperventilate by means of respiratory compensation and hence patient will have a lowered PCO_2.

Barrett K, Barman S, Boitano S, and Brooks HL (2009) *Ganong's Review of Medical Physiology*, 23rd edition. USA: McGraw-Hill.

10 Anaemia:

a **True** Conventionally anaemia is defined as a haemoglobin level of <13 g/dl in the male and <12 g/dl in the female. The thresholds for treating anaemia have changed: a patient is unlikely to be transfused until the haemoglobin is less than 7 g/dl, unless there are specific indications, for example cardiovascular disease. This change in practice is the result of trials comparing liberal and restrictive transfusion triggers.

b **True** A common cause of iron deficiency anaemia is chronic blood loss. This is a normochromic, normocytic anaemia and the patient normally compensates well to the chronic development of anaemia.

c **True** Chronic inflammatory disorders are associated with anaemia. Suppression of red cell production, non-steroidal anti-inflammatory drug (NSAID)-related blood loss, and bone marrow depression have all been suggested as possible causes of anaemia.

d **True** The anaemia associated with hypothyroidism is thought to be secondary to inadequate stimulation of red cell development in the bone marrow. When thyroid supplements are given the anaemia usually resolves.

e **True** In chronic renal failure (CRF) there is decreased erythropoietin production by the kidney leading to anaemia. Patients with CRF may have haemoglobin levels as low as 6–8 g/dl. The introduction of recombinant erythropoietin (EPO) has drastically changed the management of chronic renal failure associated anaemia.

Allman K and Wilson I. (2006) *Oxford Handbook of Anaesthesia*, 2nd edition. USA: Oxford University Press.

Pocock G and Richards C (2004) *Human Physiology: The basis of medicine*, 3rd edition. Oxford: Oxford University Press.

11 Cyanosis:

a **False** Hypercarbia produces peripheral vasodilation and warm pink skin. Cyanosis will only be a feature in the presence of hypoxia and reduced haemoglobin.

b **False** An anaemic patient does not have sufficient haemoglobin to produce cyanosis.

c **False** When arterial blood contains greater than 5 g/dl of reduced haemoglobin, cyanosis will be evident. It is for this reason that an anaemic patient will not exhibit cyanosis.

d **True** When the red cell count is high as in this condition, there is greater incidence of cyanosis even under otherwise normal conditions.

e **False** The pathology in cyanide poisoning is the inability of tissues to take up the oxygen from the haemoglobin and therefore the patient exhibits a remarkably healthy colour.

Barrett K, Barman S, Boitano S, and Brooks HL (2009) *Ganong's Review of Medical Physiology*, 23rd edition. USA: McGraw-Hill.

12 Regarding the speed of diffusion of air, oxygen, carbon dioxide, nitrogen, and nitrous oxide through the alveolus:

a **False** Oxygen diffuses slower than carbon dioxide but faster than the other gases.
b **False** Carbon dioxide diffuses across the alveolus 20 times faster than oxygen and all the other gases.
c **True** Nitrous oxide diffuses slower than oxygen and carbon dioxide, but faster than nitrogen. In the presence of pneumothorax, nitrous oxide is contraindicated (which includes Entonox®), because it can diffuse into an air-filled cavity faster than nitrogen can come out, thus increasing the size of the pneumothorax.
d **True** Nitrogen diffuses slower than all of the other gases.
e **False** Air diffuses slower than carbon dioxide, oxygen, and nitrous oxide but diffuses faster than nitrogen. Air contains oxygen and nitrogen and thus diffuses faster than nitrogen alone.

Guyton A and Hall J (2000) *Textbook of Medical Physiology*, 10th edition. Philadelphia: WB Saunders.

13 Increasing the intrathoracic pressure to 40 cmH_2O in a normal person produces the following changes initially:

a **False** The increase in intrathoracic pressure expels blood from the thoracic vessels causing an initial transient rise in blood pressure.
b **True** Peripheral resistance will show a corresponding decrease as blood pressure increases.
c **True** The sudden emptying of the thoracic vessels will produce a sudden increase in blood volume and therefore stroke volume will increase.
d **False** Initially as the blood pressure rises suddenly there is a corresponding decrease in heart rate. Later when the blood pressure begins to fall as a result of reduced venous return there will be an increase in heart rate.
e **True** The initial increase in blood pressure will cause an increase in baroreceptor rate of discharge, initiating the baroreceptor reflex, which acts to lower the blood pressure and heart rate.

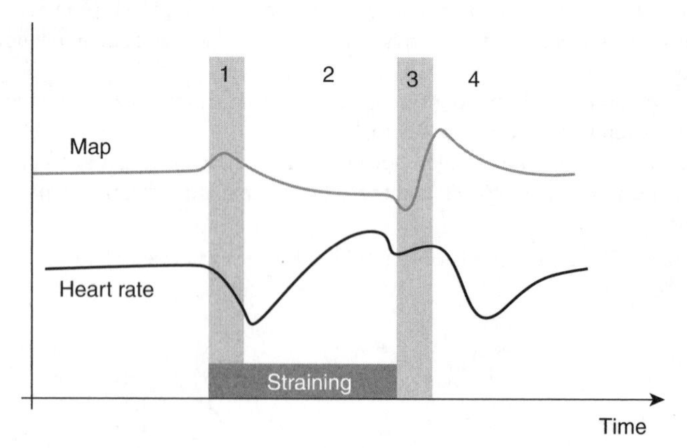

Figure 1.4 The Valsalva manoeuvre.
Reproduced with kind permission from Kevin K and Spoors C (2009) *Training in Anaesthesia*. New York: Oxford University Press.

Barrett K, Barman S, Boitano S, and Brooks HL (2009) *Ganong's Review of Medical Physiology*, 23rd edition. USA: McGraw-Hill.
Kevin K and Spoors C (2009) *Training in Anaesthesia*. New York: Oxford University Press.

14 Hyperventilation:

a **False** Respiratory alkalosis predominates. Arterial pH can return to normal only when the metabolic compensation begins.

b **True** The ionized calcium levels fall and can cause tetany.

c **False** The usual response is metabolic acidosis.

d **False** Standard bicarbonate is a derived value, after correcting the PCO_2 to normal levels and is therefore is not affected.

e **False** Hyperventilation can decrease cardiac output but because of the increase in peripheral vascular resistance, blood pressure remains the same or slightly elevated.

Barrett K, Barman S, Boitano S, and Brooks HL (2009) *Ganong's Review of Medical Physiology*, 23rd edition. USA: McGraw-Hill.

15 At high altitude:

a **True** Oxygen tension (partial pressure) is reduced. At 5791 m (19 000 ft), barometric pressure is halved, giving an inspired PO_2 of 9 kPa (50.2 kPa – 6 kPa) × 0.2093 rather than the PO_2 of 20 kPa at sea level (101 kPa – 6 kPa) × 0.2093. Partial pressure of inspired gas is equal to barometric pressure minus water vapour pressure multiplied by the concentration of the gas.

b **False** Oxygen percentage remains the same.

c **False** Density of the air is reduced.

d **True** If a person at altitude breathes at a normal rate they will have a normal $PaCO_2$. The use of the alveolar gas equation shows that their PAO_2 will be low. Loss of consciousness would occur. In order to prevent this there is a compensatory tachypnoea at altitude to decrease the $PaCO_2$ so that the PAO_2 rises.

e **True** There is hypoxic pulmonary vasoconstriction in response to hypoxia, which leads to an increase in the pulmonary arterial pressure.

Pinnock C, Lin T, and Smith T (2002) *Fundamentals of Anaesthesia*, 2nd edition. New York: Cambridge University Press.

16 Alveolar–arterial oxygen difference:

a **True** The standard difference of 0.5–1 kPa is increased if there is venous admixture (shunt).

b **True** A figure of <2 kPa is normal when breathing air, increasing to 4 kPa in the elderly. When breathing 100% O_2 the A–a difference increases to 15 kPa as the shunt component is not corrected.

c **True** Under general anaesthesia the physiological shunt increases to 7–11% and hence the alveolar–arterial oxygen difference increases.

d **True** Hypovolaemia increases the shunt with similar results.

e **False** The gradient remains the same.

Barrett K, Barman S, Boitano S, and Brooks HL (2009) *Ganong's Review of Medical Physiology*, 23rd edition. USA: McGraw-Hill.

17 Cardiac index:

a **False** It is body size and not weight that is important.

b **False** Peripheral resistance does not feature in calculation of the cardiac index.

c **False** Cardiac index (CI) is given by:

$$\text{CI (l/min/m}^2\text{)} = \frac{\text{CO (l/min)}}{\text{BSA (m}^2\text{)}}$$

where CO is cardiac output and BSA is body surface area.

d **False** Gender is irrelevant as the cardiac index is corrected for body surface area.

e **False** Cardiac index has the units l/min/m^2. The average 70 kg adult has a BSA of 1.7 m^2, giving a cardiac index of 3–3.5 l/min/m^2.

Barrett K, Barman S, Boitano S, and Brooks HL (2009) *Ganong's Review of Medical Physiology*, 23rd edition. USA: McGraw-Hill.

18 With respect to the lungs:

a **True** Both chest wall and lungs have elastic properties that interact to provide an overall value for total compliance. This would be lost when the chest is open and lung exposed.

b **True** In a normal individual the perfusion (alveolar blood flow) is equal to the alveolar ventilation at rest, V/Q = 1.

c **False** The diffusing capacity is 20 ml/min/mmHg at rest (range 17–25) and is equal to the volume of substance transferred across the alveoli per minute per unit alveolar pressure.

d **True** In the supine position the total blood volume in the pulmonary reservoir increases by approximately 400 ml. This explains the symptom of orthopnoea in a person with congestive cardiac failure.

e **True** As the lungs receive all of the cardiac output, they are well placed to undertake a metabolic function. A number of substances are metabolized by the lungs, including angiotensin I, bradykinin, leukotrienes, 5HT and prostaglandins E_2 and $F_{2\alpha}$.

Barrett K, Barman S, Boitano S, and Brooks HL (2009) *Ganong's Review of Medical Physiology*, 23rd edition. USA: McGraw-Hill.

Pinnock C, Lin T, and Smith T (2002) *Fundamentals of Anaesthesia*, 2nd edition. New York: Cambridge University Press.

19 Basal metabolic rate (BMR):

a **False** It is 2000 kcal in an average size individual.

b **False** It is lower in females than in males at all ages.

c **False** The basal metabolic rate is lower in the tropics and also in Asia.

d **True** The BMR is not necessarily at the minimum rate during sleep, the metabolic rate my decrease even further in other situations.

e **True** The BMR of a man aged 30 and age 60 is 39.3 kcal/cm^2/hour and 35.5 kcal/cm^2/hour, respectively.

Barrett K, Barman S, Boitano S, and Brooks HL (2009) *Ganong's Review of Medical Physiology*, 23rd edition. USA: McGraw-Hill.

Pinnock C, Lin T, and Smith T (2002) *Fundamentals of Anaesthesia*, 2nd edition. New York: Cambridge University Press.

20 Factors leading to increased insulin secretion include:

a **False** Only agents which are predominantly beta-adrenergic stimulants will increase insulin secretion.

b **True** As well as promoting glycogenolysis and gluconeogenesis, glucagon stimulates secretion of growth hormone, insulin, and somatostatin.

c **False** It is shown that phenytoin depresses insulin secretion.

d **False** Beta blockers inhibit insulin secretion *in vitro* but not *in vivo*. They also block the adrenergic response to hypoglycaemia, masking the signs and increasing the risk of hypoglycaemic coma. Diabetic patients prescribed beta blockers must be warned specifically of this effect.

e) **True** Sulphonylureas stimulate insulin secretion and hence exert a hypoglycaemic action.

Barrett K, Barman S, Boitano S, and Brooks HL (2009) *Ganong's Review of Medical Physiology*, 23rd edition. USA: McGraw-Hill.

Yentis S, Hirsh N, and Smith G (2003) *Anaesthesia and Intensive Care A to Z*, 3rd edition. London: Butterworth-Heinemann.

21 Features of restrictive lung disorders include:

a **False** Although both the FEV_1 and forced vital capacity (FVC) may be reduced, the FEV_1:FVC ratio is normal or even increased.

b **True** Loss of lung volumes as a whole will reduce the PEFR.

c **False** The transfer factor is only decreased in diseases such as sarcoidosis and beryllium poisoning which cause fibrosis of the alveolar walls and produce alveolar–capillary block.

d **False** As the entire lung volume is reduced, the residual volume will be reduced accordingly.

e **False** The total lung capacity will also be reduced, as will all the lung volumes.

Table 1.5 Common medical conditions and lung function testing

	FEV_1	FVC	FEV_1/FVC	Bronchodilator response	MMEF	RV	K_{CO}
Asthma	Normal or ↓	Normal or ↓	Normal or ↓	Yes	Normal or ↓	Normal	Normal
Small airways disease	Reduced	Normal or ↓	↓	Yes	↓	↑	Normal
Emphysema	Reduced	Normal or ↓	↓	No	↓	↑	↓
Pulmonary fibrosis	Normal or ↓	↓	↑	No	Normal or ↓	↓	↓
Obesity	Normal or ↓	Normal or ↓	Normal or ↑	No	Normal	↓	Normal
Kyphoscoliosis	Normal or ↓	↓	↑	No	Normal	↓	Normal
Respiratory muscle disease	Normal or ↓	↓	↑	No	Normal	↓	Normal
Pneumonectomy	↓	↓	Normal	No	Normal	↓	Normal

Barrett K, Barman S, Boitano S, and Brooks HL (2009) *Ganong's Review of Medical Physiology*, 23rd edition. USA: McGraw-Hill.
Kevin K and Spoors C (2009) *Training in Anaesthesia*. New York: Oxford University Press.

22 Surfactant:

a **True** By lowering surface tension the surfactant minimizes the tendency of the small alveoli to collapse and stabilizes the alveolar structure.
b **True** It increases the compliance by reducing the work required to inflate the alveoli.
c **False** Surfactant decreases the amount of alveolar fluid and thus helps to keep the alveoli dry.
d **True** Without surfactant the pressure required is about 3 kPa, just to prevent collapse of the alveoli and even more to expand them.
e **False** Surfactant production begins at 24 weeks' gestation. Surfactant production is usually insufficient in a premature infant and may lead to neonatal acute respiratory distress syndrome. A period of continuous positive airway pressure for three to seven days may be required until surfactant production is sufficient.

Barrett K, Barman S, Boitano S, and Brooks HL (2009) *Ganong's Review of Medical Physiology*, 23rd edition. USA: McGraw-Hill.
Yentis S, Hirsh N, and Smith G (2003) *Anaesthesia and Intensive Care A to Z*, 3rd edition. London: Butterworth-Heinemann.

23 Airway resistance:

a **True** The body plethysmograph is only available in specialist centres and is not routinely used.
b **True** Peak flow measurement is an easy and reliable bed side test. Normal values are age, sex, and height dependent. PEFR of 500–600 l/min is normal in average adults. Reference tables are available.
c **False** The pneumotachograph alone measures flow rate. If it is combined with readings from a body plethysmograph airway resistance can be measured.
d **False** Expiratory spasm is the predominant feature of bronchial asthma. Resistance to airflow is greater during expiration than during inspiration. This is the main cause of air trapping leading to spontaneous pneumothorax in severe asthma.
e **False** In a normal man the flow pattern is laminar in the lower respiratory tract because of the lower airway resistance.

Guyton A and Hall J (2000) *Textbook of Medical Physiology*, 10th edition. Philadelphia: WB Saunders.

24 Compensatory measures in response to metabolic acidosis include:

a **True** Change in pH acts on peripheral chemoreceptors stimulating respiration so that carbon dioxide falls. Buffering of the acid by HCO_3^- produces H_2CO_3, which is broken down to H_2O and CO_2 and is also eliminated by the lungs.
b **True** Lowering of the PCO_2 moves the reaction:
$$CO_2 + H_2O \leftrightarrow H_2CO_3 \leftrightarrow H^+ + HCO_3^-$$
towards the left, reducing the H^+ but also lowering the plasma HCO_3^-.
c **True** Sodium ions are used to buffer the hydrogen ions. They form NaH_2CO_3 and elimination of acid continues.
d **False** NH_3 ions are also used to buffer the H^+ ions and hence excretion is increased.
e **False** Metabolic acidosis is associated with hyperkalaemia. H^+ ion secretion leads to K^+ retention therefore levels increase.

Barrett K, Barman S, Boitano S, and Brooks HL (2009) *Ganong's Review of Medical Physiology*, 23rd edition. USA: McGraw-Hill.

25 Excessive secretion of mineralocorticoids:

- a **False** Excess mineralocorticoids increase potassium secretion from the distal convoluted tubule into the urine causing hypokalaemia.
- b **True** Aldosterone secretion stimulates active reabsorption of sodium ions from the distal convoluted tubule and into the blood. Water is then passively reabsorbed along with the sodium causing an increase in the circulating volume.
- c **False** Urine sodium secretion is reduced.
- d **True** Tubular secretion of hydrogen ions is enhanced leading to a metabolic alkalosis.
- e **False** Glucose metabolism is not affected. Glucocorticoids rather than mineralocorticoids affect glucose metabolism.

Barrett K, Barman S, Boitano S, and Brooks HL (2009) *Ganong's Review of Medical Physiology*, 23rd edition. USA: McGraw-Hill.
Pinnock C, Lin T, and Smith T (2002) *Fundamentals of Anaesthesia*, 2nd edition. New York: Cambridge University Press.

26 Antidiuretic hormone:

- a **False** ADH or vasopressin is produced by the supraoptic nucleus of the hypothalamus and stored in the posterior pituitary gland before being released in response to stimuli.
- b **False** The absorption in the proximal tubules is not dependent on ADH.
- c **True** ADH increases distal convoluted tubule water reabsorption, but this is not the main site of action.
- d **True** ADH increases the collecting duct permeability to water this is its main site of action.
- e **True** ADH action produces a small volume of concentrated urine (high urine osmolality).

Barrett K, Barman S, Boitano S, and Brooks HL (2009) *Ganong's Review of Medical Physiology*, 23rd edition. USA: McGraw-Hill.
Pinnock C, Lin T, and Smith T (2002) *Fundamentals of Anaesthesia*, 2nd edition. New York: Cambridge University Press.

27 Cardiac output:

- a **True** Cardiac output = stroke volume × heart rate.
- b **True** By full term pregnancy the cardiac output is increased by 40%.
- c **False** Contrary to popular belief there is no change.
- d **True** Standing or sitting from a lying down position can decrease the cardiac output by 20–30%. This is a significant decrease for patients with coexisting cardiovascular disease and can lead to syncope.
- e **False** Adrenaline (epinephrine) leads to an increase in cardiac output via its effect on beta 1 receptors.

Barrett K, Barman S, Boitano S, and Brooks HL (2009) *Ganong's Review of Medical Physiology*, 23rd edition. USA: McGraw-Hill.

28 Anatomical dead space:

a **True** It is equivalent to the conducting airways that do not take part in gas exchange (trachea, main bronchi up to the bronchioles) and it is approximately 2–3 ml/kg. Anatomical dead space is 150 ml for a 70 kg person.

b **True** Anatomical dead space is reduced in the sitting or lying position.

c **True** Extending the neck and protruding the jaw causes an increase volume of air in the conducting airways therefore increases dead space.

d **True** Atropine produces bronchodilation and hence increases the dead space.

e **True** The normal ratio of dead space to tidal volume is 0.2:0.35 during resting breathing. Normal tidal volume is 500 ml, normal dead space is 150 ml. During rapid shallow breathing, despite normal minute ventilation, alveolar ventilation is reduced because a greater proportion of the tidal volume is the dead space.

Aitkenhead A and Smith G (2008) *Textbook of Anaesthesia*, 5th edition. Edinburgh: Churchill Livingstone.

29 Physiological dead space:

a **True** Physiological dead space can be calculated using the Bohr equation:

$$\frac{V_D}{V_T} = \frac{PaCO_2 - P_ECO_2}{P_aCO_2}$$

where V_D = dead space V_T = tidal volume $PaCO_2$ = arterial PCO_2 and P_ECO_2 = expired PCO_2

Physiological dead space is increased in respiratory disease and under anaesthesia.

b **True** Bohr's method measures the volume of lung that does not eliminate carbon dioxide

c **True** The normal ratio of dead space to tidal volume is 0.2:0.35 during normal resting breathing.

d **True** Other factors that increase the dead space include old age, hypotension, haemorrhage, and general anaesthesia.

e **True** The physiological dead space is the sum of anatomical and alveolar dead space (alveoli ventilated but not perfused). In healthy individuals this is negligible and both dead spaces can be assumed to be the same.

Aitkenhead A and Smith G (2008) *Textbook of Anaesthesia*, 5th edition. Edinburgh: Churchill Livingstone.
West J (2004) *Respiratory Physiology*, 7th edition. Philadelphia: Lippincott Williams and Wilkins.

30 Left atrial pressure

a **False** It is 2–5 mmHg. The right atrial pressure is 0–2 mmHg.

b **True** PCWP is measured with a pulmonary artery catheter when it occludes a pulmonary vessel. The catheter tip is then separated from the left atrium by a continuous column of blood. Thus the PCWP normally approximates to the left atrial pressure.

c **False** Usually a pressure >25 mmHg indicates left heart failure.

d **True** In heart failure the right-sided pressures do not accurately reflect the filling status and so the PCWP may be a more useful guide. However, the use of the pulmonary artery catheter outside specialist centres has declined in favour of less invasive means such as the oesophageal Doppler monitor.

e **True** The initial rise in left atrial pressure up-to 7–8 mmHg has no noticeable effects on pulmonary circulation because initially this increase merely expands the pulmonary venules and opens up more capillaries. Further increases in left atrial pressure cause almost equally great increases in pulmonary artery pressure, thus placing the same pressure load on the right heart. When the pressure reaches 30 mmHg or more, pulmonary oedema is likely.

Barrett K, Barman S, Boitano S, and Brooks HL (2009) *Ganong's Review of Medical Physiology*, 23rd edition. USA: McGraw-Hill.

30 Left atrial pressure

False.

chapter 2

PHARMACOLOGY

QUESTIONS

1 Non-depolarizing neuromuscular blocking agents may be potentiated by:

a Hypermagnesaemia
b Streptomycin
c Gentamicin
d Acetylcholinesterase
e Inhalational agents

2 Match the following intravenous (IV) fluids with their corresponding pH:

a	NaCl 0.9%	4.0
b	Hartmann's solution (Ringer's lactate)	5.0
c	Dextrose	6.5
d	Sodium bicarbonate 8.4%	8.0
e	Gelofusine®	7.4

3 Bupivacaine:

a Requires higher drug concentration in plasma for a toxic effect compared to lidocaine (lignocaine)
b Has a safe upper dose limit of 2 mg/kg
c When used for a nerve block may produce effects lasting greater than eight hours
d Duration of action is increased by the addition of adrenaline (epinephrine)
e Is excreted unchanged by the kidneys

4 Heparin:

a Is so called because it was first extracted from the liver
b Has a half-life of 40–90 minutes
c Is given in a dose of 24 000–48 000 units over 24 hours in deep vein thrombosis (DVT)
d Is commercially extracted from the sperm of salmon and various other fish
e Can be reversed by giving vitamin K

5 Suxamethonium:

a Raises intraocular pressure
b May produce a rise of 2–3 mmol of potassium in susceptible individuals
c Action is prolonged by tetrahydroaminacrine
d May produce prolonged neuromuscular blockade in pregnancy
e With higher doses, the duration of relaxation is increased

6 Pancuronium:

a Has a steroid nucleus
b Dose is 0.1–0.5 mg/kg
c Produces significant histamine release
d Has a duration of action of 30–45 minutes
e Is contraindicated in phaeochromocytoma

7 Local anaesthetic drugs:

a Act by reducing the resting permeability of the nerve membrane
b Act efficiently at low pH
c Which are carbonated have a longer duration of action
d Will produce convulsions before cardiovascular depression
e May be used during induction of anaesthesia to produce cardiac stability in patients with ischaemic heart disease

8 Drugs that should be avoided in patients taking monoamine oxidase inhibitors (MAOIs) include:

a Pethidine
b Tramadol
c Ephedrine
d Cocaine
e Morphine

9 Adrenergic neurone blocking drugs:

a Act mainly on the postganglionic adrenergic nerve fibres
b May produce a 'blocked Valsalva' response
c Produce hypotension
d Do not interfere with renal blood flow
e May interfere with estimation of urinary catecholamines

10 The following drugs act on both alpha and beta receptors:

a Isoprenaline
b Labetalol
c Noradrenaline (norepinephrine)
d Metaraminol
e Terbutaline

11 Minimum alveolar concentration (MAC):

a Is the concentration of an anaesthetic agent required to suppress reflex movements to skin incision in the subjects studied
b Correlates well with the blood/gas coefficient
c Can be achieved quicker with sevoflurane than isoflurane
d Is directly proportional to an agent's potency
e Of sevoflurane is the lowest of the inhalational agents

12 Atropine:

- a Is a more potent antisialogogue than hyoscine
- b May initially produce vagal stimulation
- c Does not cross the placenta
- d Appears in small amounts in sweat and breast milk
- e Is mainly excreted by the kidneys

13 Digoxin:

- a Decreases the refractory period of the myocardium
- b Improves myocardial contractility
- c Undergoes renal excretion
- d Has a small therapeutic:toxic ratio
- e May increase myocardial irritability

14 Miosis is produced by the following:

- a Pilocarpine
- b Timolol
- c Homatropine
- d Nicotine
- e Alcohol

15 Methaemoglobinaemia may be seen with:

- a Sodium nitrite
- b Methylene blue
- c Lidocaine (lignocaine)
- d Prilocaine
- e Mepivacaine

16 Oral anticoagulants:

- a Are active both *in vivo* and *in vitro*
- b Exert their action after a latent period of two to four hours
- c Increase both the bleeding and clotting times
- d Are potentiated by barbiturates
- e Action can be reversed with protamine

17 The action of suxamethonium may be prolonged by:

- a Ecothiopate
- b Cyclophosphamide
- c Kwashiorkor
- d Trimetaphan
- e Liver failure

18 Uterine action is depressed by:

a Terbutaline
b GTN
c Isoprenaline
d Noradrenaline (norepinephrine)
e Ketamine

19 Propofol:

a Is chemically 2,6-diisopropylphenol
b Is a hydrophilic substance
c Plasma protein binding is approximately 50%
d Gives a quicker recovery than after thiopental (thiopentone)
e Has a short duration of action mainly due to redistribution

20 Ketamine:

a Is a phencyclidine derivative
b Blocks *N*-methyl-D-aspartate (NMDA) receptors
c Can only be administered IV
d Is useful as an adjunct to IV induction in asthmatic people
e Increases intracranial pressure

21 Drugs that cross the blood–brain barrier include:

a Suxamethonium
b Atropine
c Tubocurarine
d Glycopyrrolate
e Hyoscine

22 Emergency treatment of severe hyperkalaemia includes:

a IV calcium
b IV insulin
c Furosemide
d Steroids
e Oral ion exchange resins

23 Nitrous oxide:

a Is manufactured by heating NH_4NO_3 to 245°C
b Its weight in the cylinder is calculated by knowing the tare weight
c Blood/gas coefficient is 0.69
d Has a critical temperature of 45°C
e Has a MAC of 90

24 Concerning drug–receptor interactions:

- a Competitive antagonism refers to a drug that binds to a receptor and prevents an agonist from binding to the same receptor.
- b A drug that causes a submaximal response is called a partial agonist
- c Tachyphylaxis describes the enhanced response to repetitive administration of a drug
- d A ligand is a protein that interferes with drug binding to a receptor
- e The maximal response a drug can produce when given in high concentrations is termed its intrinsic activity

25 Regarding drug interactions:

- a An additive effect is two drugs working together to produce an effect that is greater than the sum of their individual effects
- b Heparin and protamine are examples of chemical incompatibility
- c Probenecid increases the activity of penicillin by decreasing its renal excretion
- d Adrenaline (epinephrine) and propranolol are competitive antagonists
- e Benzodiazepines displace phenytoin from plasma protein binding sites

26 Drugs producing bronchodilation include:

- a Hyoscine
- b Ipratropium bromide
- c Adrenaline (epinephrine)
- d Muscarine
- e Promethazine

27 Hyperglycaemia may be associated with:

- a Isoprenaline infusion
- b Epidural anaesthesia with bupivacaine
- c Thiopental (thiopentone)
- d Ketamine
- e Enflurane

28 Drugs increasing cerebral blood flow include:

- a Halothane
- b Enflurane
- c Ketamine
- d Propofol
- e Thiopental (thiopentone)

29 Heparin exerts its anticoagulant action by:

- a Antithromboplastic action
- b Prevention of thrombin conversion
- c Prevention of fibrin formation
- d Reducing platelet adhesiveness
- e Facilitation of resolution of clots

30 Anaesthetic drugs that are safe in dystrophia myotonica include:

a Suxamethonium
b Propofol infusion for maintenance
c Thiopental (thiopentone) infusion
d Opiate analgesia in standard doses
e Anticholinesterases

chapter 2

PHARMACOLOGY

ANSWERS

1 Non-depolarizing neuromuscular blocking agents may be potentiated by:

- a **True** Acetylcholine release decreases as magnesium competes with calcium and stabilizes the post-junctional membrane.
- b **True** This was first noticed in the days when large quantities of streptomycin powder were placed in the spinal column or chest cavity after surgery for tuberculosis. When such patients were unable to breathe adequately, the association between the relaxants and the antibiotic was discovered. Other antibiotics prolonging neuromuscular blocking drug action include polymyxins and tetracycline.
- c **True** Aminoglycosides are associated with prolonged action of neuromuscular blocking drugs.
- d **True** Acetylcholinesterase is the enzyme that destroys acetylcholine at the nerve endings, and hence it will prolong the action of non-depolarizing muscle relaxants.
- e **True** Inhalational anaesthetic agents cause depression of transmitter release at the neuromuscular junction. However, current inhalational agents do not potentiate relaxants to the same extent as halothane or diethyl ether.

Peck T, Hill S, and Williams M (2004) *Pharmacology for Anaesthesia and Intensive Care*, 2nd edition. Cambridge: Cambridge University Press.

2 Match the following IV fluids with their corresponding pH:

- a **False** The pH of 0.9% saline is 5.0.
- b **False** Hartmann's solution or Ringer's lactate has a pH of 6.0.
- c **False** Dextrose 5% and 10% solutions have a pH of 4.0. They are one of the most acidic solutions administered and therefore greater caution is needed before any additives are mixed with them.
- d **True** It is alkaline and injection into a small peripheral vein may cause irritation.
- e **True** It has the same pH as plasma under normal conditions.

Aitkenhead A and Smith G (2008) *Textbook of Anaesthesia*, 5th edition. Edinburgh: Churchill Livingstone.

3 Bupivacaine:

a **False** The toxic plasma concentration for lidocaine (lignocaine) is 5 μg/ml whereas for bupivacaine it is 2–4 μg/ml.
b **True** The safe upper limit for bupivacaine is 2 mg/kg.
c **True** Duration varies according to the type of nerve block, for example brachial plexus blocks may last up to 12 hours.
d **False** Bupivacaine exhibits high binding to plasma proteins. Addition of adrenaline (ephedrine) does not increase its duration of action, unlike lidocaine.
e **False** Only 5% of the injected bupivacaine appears in the urine as the *N*-dealkylated metabolite. The rest is metabolized in the liver by dealkylation to pipecolic acid and pipecolylxylidine.

Aitkenhead A and Smith G (2008) *Textbook of Anaesthesia*, 5th edition. Edinburgh: Churchill Livingstone.
Peck T, Hill S, and Williams M (2004) *Pharmacology for Anaesthesia and Intensive Care*, 2nd edition. Cambridge: Cambridge University Press.

4 Heparin:

a **True** Heparin is named as it was first extracted from canine liver. (*Hepar* is Greek for liver.)
b **True** The action is terminated within two hours. This should be borne in mind when discontinuing heparin prior to surgery.
c **True** In moderate DVT, a dose of 1000 units per hour over 24 hours is considered suitable.
d **False** It is protamine that is extracted from the sperm of salmon and other fish.
e **False** Vitamin K is used for reversal of warfarin.

Peck T, Hill S, and Williams M (2004) *Pharmacology for Anaesthesia and Intensive Care*, 2nd edition. Cambridge: Cambridge University Press.

5 Suxamethonium:

a **True** The intraocular pressure rises with administration of suxamethonium. This results from contraction of extraocular muscles applying pressure to the orbit. This is of extreme importance in patients with open eye injuries, where the vitreous might be completely extruded resulting in blindness.
b **True** Although the rise is usually no more than 0.5 mmol, it may be greater in susceptible patients, for example following burns, spinal cord injury and many muscle disorders.
c **True** Tetrahydroaminocrine (Tacrine) was originally used to prolong the action of suxamethonium and to decrease muscle pains following its administration.
d **True** Pseudocholinesterase quantity is reduced in pregnancy and therefore prolongation of action can occur.
e **False** Unlike the non-depolarizing relaxants, higher doses of suxamethonium do not increase the duration of action but increase the extent of relaxation.

Peck T, Hill S, and Williams M (2004) *Pharmacology for Anaesthesia and Intensive Care*, 2nd edition. Cambridge: Cambridge University Press.

6 Pancuronium:

a **True** It is a bis quaternary aminosteroid.
b **False** The usual initial dose is 0.05–0.1 mg/kg.
c **False** Is does not cause significant histamine release. Historically, it was preferable to use pancuronium instead of tubocurarine in the anaesthetic management of phaeochromocytoma, because the significant release of histamine by the latter predisposes to a hypertensive episode (secondary to increased catecholamine secretion).
d **False** The normal duration of action is 45–120 minutes.
e **False** A significant tachycardia is observed with the first (loading) dose of pancuronium. This is believed to be due to rapid depletion of adrenaline (epinephrine) and noradrenaline (norepinephrine) from nerve endings. A similar response is not seen with subsequent doses, which are about 25% of the original dose. Although it is no longer in regular use, specialized cardiovascular centres still use pancuronium because of the cardiovascular stability it provides.

Aitkenhead A and Smith G (2008) *Textbook of Anaesthesia*, 5th edition. Edinburgh: Churchill Livingstone.

7 Local anaesthetic drugs:

a **True** A nerve impulse cannot be propagated unless the sodium pump can cause the reversal of the ionic gradient across the cell membrane.
b **False** Local anaesthetics cannot work efficiently in an acid medium as this decreases the proportion of the drug in the un-ionized state.
c **False** Carbonated local anaesthetic agents have a faster onset of action because of easy access to bicarbonate ions. The carbon dioxide already available in the mixture is converted to bicarbonate when it is injected into the site. The duration of action, however, is the same as or shorter than the non-carbonated versions.
d **True** Although this is debated currently, it appears that convulsions (despite being rare) are seen more frequently than complete cardiovascular collapse. With bupivacaine, a blood level of 4 μg/ml is considered the limit above which adverse effects may be observed, and there are more reported cases of convulsions than cardiovascular collapse.
e **True** Plain lidocaine (lignocaine) in a 1 mg/kg dose has been used to reduce cardiovascular irritability and also as a means of suppressing the autonomic response to laryngoscopy and intubation.

Aitkenhead A and Smith G (2008) *Textbook of Anaesthesia*, 5th edition. Edinburgh: Churchill Livingstone.

8 Drugs that should be avoided in patients taking monoamine oxidase inhibitors (MAOIs) include:

a **True** Pethidine decreases the uptake of 5-hydroxytryptamine (5-HT; serotonin) from nerve endings. When given with MAOIs it can produce excessive levels of 5HT and hypertension, pyrexia, tachycardia, and convulsions, or 'serotonin syndrome'.

b **True** Tramadol also increases 5HT release.

c **True** Sympathomimetic drugs, especially indirectly acting drugs such as ephedrine and metaraminol, cause an exaggerated hypertensive response.

d **True** Cocaine inhibits monoamine oxidase and also prevents the uptake of noradrenaline (norepinephrine).

e **False** Morphine is considered safe to use in patients taking MAOIs. Some have reported no problems with fentanyl, but as it is derived from pethidine, others prefer to avoid its use. Pentazocine has also been used in the past.

Yentis S, Hirsh N, and Smith G (2003) *Anaesthesia and Intensive Care A to Z*, 3rd edition. London: Butterworth-Heinemann.

9 Adrenergic neurone blocking drugs:

a **True** They are believed to prevent release or reuptake of noradrenaline (norepinephrine) in the postganglionic adrenergic neurone.

b **True** A 'blocked Valsalva' can be the result of treatment with these drugs because they disrupt one limb of the reflex arc, thus preventing a normal baroreceptor response to hypotension.

c **True** Inhibition of noradrenaline (norepinephrine) release produces hypotension, which is the main action of these drugs.

d **False** Renal circulation is reduced.

e **True** Breakdown products of noradrenaline (norepinephrine) will initially increase in the urine as it is displaced from its binding sites.

Rang H, Dale M, and Ritter J (2000) *Rang and Dales' Pharmacology*, 6th edition. Edinburgh: Churchill Livingstone.

10 The following drugs act on both alpha and beta receptors:

a **False** Isoprenaline is a pure beta agonist at beta 1 and beta 2 receptors.

b **True** Labetalol is an alpha and beta blocker which is used as an infusion for hypotensive anaesthesia and orally in the treatment of severe hypertension and pre-eclampsia.

c **True** Although noradrenaline (norepinephrine) predominantly stimulates α receptors, it does exhibit some effect on β_1 receptors.

d **True** Metaraminol has predominantly alpha action but also has some beta adrenoceptor activity. It also has an indirect action via adrenaline (epinephrine) and noradrenaline (norepinephrine) release.

e **False** It is a beta receptor agonist.

Peck T, Hill S, and Williams M (2004) *Pharmacology for Anaesthesia and Intensive Care*, 2nd edition. Cambridge: Cambridge University Press.

11 Minimum alveolar concentration (MAC):

a **False** It is the minimum alveolar concentration of an inhalational agent to suppress response to skin incision in 50% of subjects studied.

b **False** The oil/gas coefficient gives an indication of potency of a given agent.

c **True** Since sevoflurane is a non-irritant, cardio-stable agent, higher concentrations (e.g. 8%) can be delivered without any cardiorespiratory problems and thereby achieve the MAC quickly. Sevoflurane is also less pungent than isoflurane so that patients tolerate breathing higher concentrations.

d **False** Agents with a lower MAC have a higher potency.

e **False** Of the currently used inhalational agents desflurane has a MAC of 6.3, sevoflurane of 2.0, and isoflurane of 1.17.

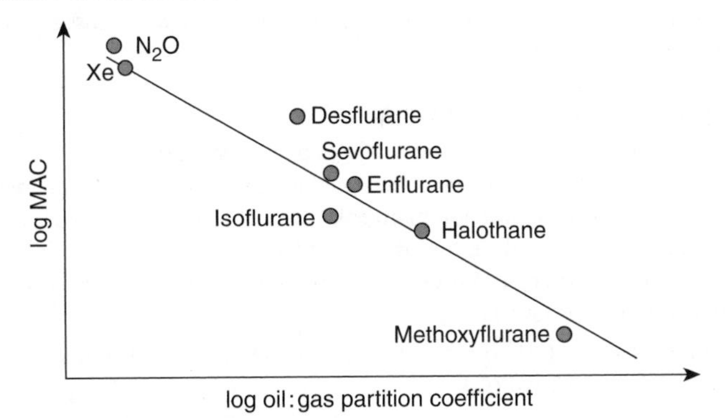

Figure 2.1 Minimum alveolar concentration (MAC) versus the oil/gas partition coefficient. Reproduced with kind permission from Kevin K and Spoors C (2009) *Training in Anaesthesia*. New York: Oxford University Press.

Aitkenhead A and Smith G (2008) *Textbook of Anaesthesia*, 5th edition. Edinburgh: Churchill Livingstone.
Kevin K and Spoors C (2009) *Training in Anaesthesia*. New York: Oxford University Press.
Pinnock C, Lin T, and Smith T (2002) *Fundamentals of Anaesthesia*, 2nd edition. New York: Cambridge University Press.

12 Atropine:

a **True** Hyoscine is an efficient antisialogogue, but it is noted more for its sedative and antiemetic effects.

b **True** In low dose, atropine may produce a paradoxical bradycardia.

c **False** All available evidence suggests that atropine crosses the placenta to a variable extent.

d **True** Atropine appears in small amounts in sweat and breast milk, although the amounts in breast milk are negligible and will not cause an effect in the neonate.

e **False** Only a small fraction is excreted unchanged in the urine.

Aitkenhead A and Smith G (2008) *Textbook of Anaesthesia*, 5th edition. Edinburgh: Churchill Livingstone.

13 Digoxin:

a **False** It increases the refractory period of the atrioventricular node, thus slowing the heart rate.
b **True** Slowing of the heart rate improves the pumping efficiency of the ventricles.
c **True** The elimination half-life of digoxin in patients with normal renal function is approximately 36 hours, which may be considerably increased in renal failure, necessitating reduction in dose.
d **True** Blood levels of 1–2.6 nmol/l can be therapeutic and toxic levels overlap the upper limit of the therapeutic level.
e **True** Ventricular ectopics, bigeminy and ventricular tachycardia are examples of the dysrhythmias associated with digoxin overdose.

Peck T, Hill S, and Williams M (2004) *Pharmacology for Anaesthesia and Intensive Care*, 2nd edition. Cambridge: Cambridge University Press.

14 Miosis is produced by the following:

a **True** It is a muscarinic agent used as eye drops in glaucoma.
b **True** It is a beta blocker and has been used for the same purpose as above.
c **False** Homatropine is a version of atropine and does not cause miosis.
d **False** Nicotine may produce the opposite effect.
e **False** Alcohol poisoning can produce an unevenly reacting pupil known as 'MacEwen pupil' but does not produce miosis.

Peck T, Hill S, and Williams M (2004) *Pharmacology for Anaesthesia and Intensive Care*, 2nd edition. Cambridge: Cambridge University Press.

15 Methaemoglobinaemia may be seen with:

a **True** Oxidizing agents or drugs such as nitrites may cause methaemoglobinaemia.
b **False** Methylene blue is used in the treatment of methaemoglobinaemia. It acts to reduce the haem group from methaemoglobin to haemoglobin.
c **False** Lidocaine (lignocaine) in clinically used doses is not implicated however, larger doses may produce methaemoglobin by affecting the metabolism in the liver.
d **True** Prilocaine has been reported to cause methaemoglobinaemia but it is usually seen when the maximum recommended dose is exceeded.
e **False** It is a longer acting agent than lidocaine and has not been implicated in methaemoglobinaemia.

Aitkenhead A and Smith G (2008) *Textbook of Anaesthesia*, 5th edition. Edinburgh: Churchill Livingstone.
Davies N and Cashman J (1999) *Lee's Synopsis of Anaesthesia*. 13th edition. Oxford: Butterworth-Heinemann.
Peck T, Hill S, and Williams M (2004) *Pharmacology for Anaesthesia and Intensive Care*, 2nd edition. Cambridge: Cambridge University Press.

16 Oral anticoagulants:

a **False** They are active only *in vivo*.

b **False** The effect takes at least 40–48 hours to develop.

c **False** Bleeding time is normally two to nine minutes and was used as a test for integrity of functioning platelets. Since oral anticoagulants interfere mainly with factors II, VII, IX, and X, they prolong the clotting time, expressed as the international normalized ratio (INR).

d **False** Barbiturates are potent enzyme induction agents and hence decrease the action of these drugs.

e **False** Protamine neutralizes the action of heparin. Vitamin K or fresh frozen plasma (FFP) is required to reverse the action of warfarin.

Peck T, Hill S, and Williams M (2004) *Pharmacology for Anaesthesia and Intensive Care*, 2nd edition. Cambridge: Cambridge University Press.
Aitkenhead A and Smith G (2008) *Textbook of Anaesthesia*, 5th edition. Edinburgh: Churchill Livingstone.

17 The action of suxamethonium may be prolonged by:

a **True** Ecothiopate is an anticholinesterase used as eye drops in glaucoma.

b **True** Patients treated with cyclophosphamide have been seen to have low pseudocholinesterase levels.

c **True** Kwashiorkor is a disease secondary to protein deficiency. Any condition that produces malnutrition may lead to low pseudocholinesterase levels.

d **True** Trimetaphan, a ganglion blocking drug used routinely in the past during controlled hypotension, has been shown to prolong the action of suxamethonium if the two are co-administered.

e **True** Liver failure will lead to derangement in the synthesis of pseudocholinesterase with similar consequences as seen in malnutrition.

Davies N and Cashman J (1999) *Lee's Synopsis of Anaesthesia*. 13th edition. Oxford: Butterworth-Heinemann.
Rang H, Dale M, and Ritter J (2000) *Rang and Dales' Pharmacology*, 6th edition. Edinburgh: Churchill Livingstone.

18 Uterine action is depressed by:

a **True** Although it is essentially used as a bronchodilator, terbutaline also decreases the tone of uterine muscle.

b **True** Glyceryl trinitrate in IV, sublingual, and topical form has been used to suppress uterine activity, although care must be taken to prevent hypotension.

c **True** All β_2 agonists have an action on the uterus. Isoprenaline has more action than orciprenaline.

d **False** Noradrenaline (norepinephrine) is predominantly an alpha agonist and does not affect uterine tone.

e **False** Ketamine actually increases uterine tone and is sometimes used for this property for anaesthesia for postpartum haemorrhage.

Peck T, Hill S, and Williams M (2004) *Pharmacology for Anaesthesia and Intensive Care*, 2nd edition. Cambridge: Cambridge University Press.

19 Propofol:

- a **True** The trade name 'Diprivan', stands for 'Di-isopropyl IV anaesthetic'.
- b **False** It is virtually insoluble in water. The original formulation was with Cremophor EL, which has now been changed to 10% soybean oil emulsion along with 1.2% purified egg phosphatide and 2.25% glycerol. Apart from being irritant to veins, Cremophor EL was implicated in sensitivity and allergic reactions.
- c **False** Protein binding is approximately 90%.
- d **True** It is rapidly metabolized in addition to redistribution and hence the rapid recovery.
- e **True** Following bolus administration, propofol has a short duration of action due to the rapid decrease in plasma concentration as it is distributed to well-perfused tissues. It also has no active metabolites.

OH

Propofol $(CH_3)_2{\cdot}CH$ — $CH{\cdot}(CH_3)_2$

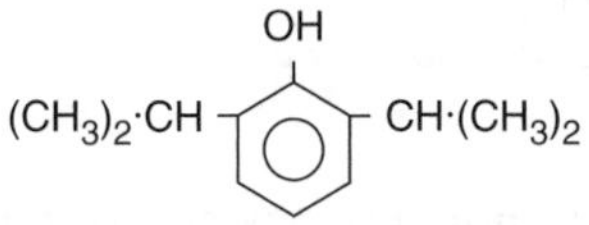

Figure 2.2 Chemical structure of propofol.
Reproduced with kind permission from Peck T, Hill S and Williams M (2008) *Pharmacology for Anaesthesia and Intensive Care*, 3rd edition, . Cambridge: Cambridge University Press.

Aitkenhead A and Smith G (2008) *Textbook of Anaesthesia*, 5th edition. Edinburgh: Churchill Livingstone.
Peck T, Hill S, and Williams M (2004) *Pharmacology for Anaesthesia and Intensive Care*, 2nd edition. Cambridge: Cambridge University Press.

20 Ketamine:

- a **True** Ketamine is also known as 'angel dust'. It is a commonly used recreational drug.
- b **True** NMDA receptors are blocked to produce the dissociative anaesthesia and the hallucinations that follow.
- c **False** Ketamine can also be used intramuscularly (IM) or orally (PO). Induction doses are 1–2 mg/kg IV and 5–10 mg/kg IM. Oral ketamine in a dose of 3–6 mg/kg has been used for premedication in children. Mixed with a soft drink it is virtually unnoticeable, making it attractive for use in children and adults with learning difficulties.
- d **True** Its smooth muscle relaxant and antihistamine properties make ketamine an ideal agent to use on its own or in conjunction with another in emergency intubation of patients with severe asthma. It may be used as a precautionary measure in asthmatic patients requiring general anaesthesia for elective surgery.
- e **True** It increases the systolic pressure and increases cerebral blood flow. It may be dangerous in patients with high intracranial pressure or those with hypertension. It is also known to increase intraocular pressure.

Peck T, Hill S, and Williams M (2004) *Pharmacology for Anaesthesia and Intensive Care*, 2nd edition. Cambridge: Cambridge University Press.
Aitkenhead A and Smith G (2008) *Textbook of Anaesthesia*, 5th edition. Edinburgh: Churchill Livingstone.

21 Drugs that cross the blood–brain barrier include:

a **False** None of the depolarizing or non-depolarizing drugs cross the blood–brain barrier because they are highly ionized agents.

b **True** Atropine can produce confusion and hallucinogenic states in the elderly. Dehydration, made worse by the drying effects of the drug, may also contribute to the restlessness of the patient.

c **False** This non-depolarizing neuromuscular blocking drug was discontinued in 1996. It was a mono quaternary alkaloid with a tertiary amine group. It is 30–50% protein bound and does not cross the blood–brain barrier.

d **False** It is this property which has led to glycopyrrolate being chosen instead of atropine, especially in the elderly.

e **True** Hyoscine can cause sedation along with its amnesic and antiemetic actions.

Aitkenhead A and Smith G (2008) *Textbook of Anaesthesia*, 5th edition. Edinburgh: Churchill Livingstone.

Davies N and Cashman J (1999) *Lee's Synopsis of Anaesthesia*, 13th edition. Oxford: Butterworth-Heinemann.

22 Emergency treatment of severe hyperkalaemia includes:

a **True** Calcium may be necessary to protect the myocardium from the negative inotropic effects of hyperkalaemia by adjusting the ionic balance.

b **True** Part of standard management is to use a dextrose and insulin infusion for quickly lowering potassium levels.

c **True** Diuretics will help to some extent in the excretion of potassium if the patient has a functioning renal system.

d **False** They do not feature in the management of hyperkalaemia.

e **True** They may be used as maintenance therapy along with other emergency measures.

Aitkenhead A and Smith G (2008) *Textbook of Anaesthesia*, 5th edition. Edinburgh: Churchill Livingstone.

23 Nitrous oxide:

a **True** This process produces nitrous oxide, along with its higher oxides, which are eliminated by passing them through various 'scrubbers'.

b **True** The empty and full weight of the cylinder is printed on the surface. It is then possible to work out the actual content of nitrous oxide in the cylinder.

c **False** It is 0.47.

d **False** The critical temperature of nitrous oxide is 36.5°C (above this temperature it cannot be liquefied with pressure alone).

e **False** It is a weak anaesthetic agent and hence has a MAC of 105. As it can be administered in high concentrations safely with oxygen, it can be used as an efficient analgesic.

Davies N and Cashman J (1999) *Lee's Synopsis of Anaesthesia*, 13th edition. Oxford: Butterworth-Heinemann.

24 Concerning drug–receptor interactions:

a **True** A competitive antagonist competes for the same receptor binding site. The effect of the antagonist may be overcome by increasing the concentration of the agonist. An example of a competitive antagonist is non-depolarizing muscle relaxants competing with acetylcholine for cholinergic binding sites at the nicotinic receptor of the neuromuscular junction.

b **True** A drug that occupies the receptors but has a less than maximum effect compared with the full agonist is termed a partial agonist. Partial agonists do not produce maximum response even when all receptors are occupied. An example is buprenorphine, a partial agonist at the mu opioid receptor.

c **False** Tachyphylaxis describes the ever-decreasing effect of a drug on repeated administration in a given time. An example is decreased response to ephedrine as noradrenaline (norepinephrine) becomes depleted.

d **False** A ligand is any substance that can bind to a receptor. They may or may not then elicit a response. Ligands may bind more than one receptor, producing different effects at each one.

e **True** The intrinsic activity of a drug, refers to what the drug does once it is bound to the receptor and is given a value from 0 to 1. An agonist has full intrinsic activity (1), an antagonist has no intrinsic activity (0), and a partial agonist has only some intrinsic activity (>0 but <1).

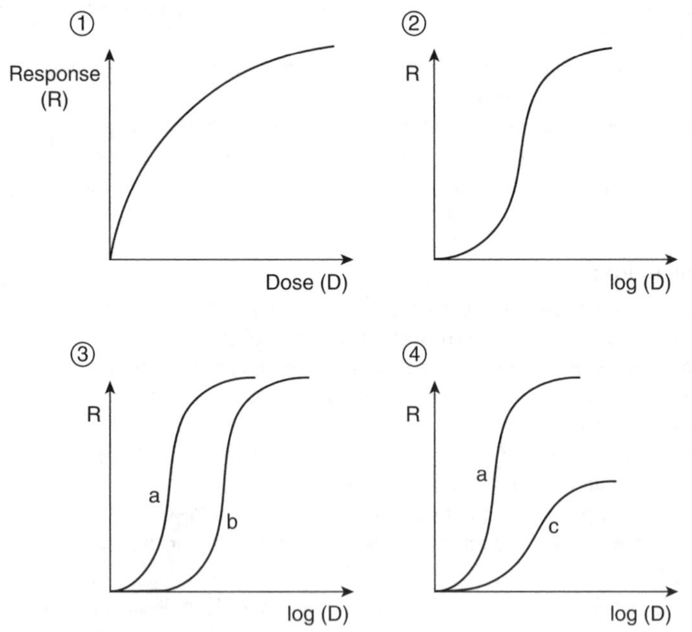

Figure 2.3 Dose–response curves:
(1) Normal agonist dose–response curve
(2) Log dose–response curve
(3) Full agonist (a) in the presence of a competitive agonist or (b) an irreversible agonist at low dose
(4) Full agonist (a) and partial agonist (c).
Taken with kind permission from Peck et al. (2008) *Pharmacology for Anaesthesia and Intensive Care*, 3rd edition. Cambridge: Cambridge University Press.

Peck T, Hill S, and Williams M (2004) *Pharmacology for Anaesthesia and Intensive Care*, 2nd edition. Cambridge: Cambridge University Press.

25 Regarding drug interactions:

a **False** An additive effect is when the product of two drugs is the sum of their individual effects.
b **True** Heparin is acidic and protamine is basic and hence they counteract each other.
c **True** This knowledge was used in the past to increase the efficacy of a given dose of penicillin.
d **True** They compete for the same receptors.
e **False** They do not compete for the same protein binding sites.

Rang H, Dale M, and Ritter J (2000) *Rang and Dales' Pharmacology*, 6th edition. Edinburgh: Churchill Livingstone.

26 Drugs producing bronchodilation include:

a **True** All antisialogogues have a bronchodilatory effect.
b **True** It is an atropine-like substance that is clinically used in patients with asthma.
c **True** Adrenaline (epinephrine) is one of the most potent bronchodilators. It is the first line treatment for bronchospasm secondary to anaphylaxis and is also used in refractory status asthmaticus.
d **False** It is a parasympathomimetic agent and would therefore produce bronchospasm.
e **True** It is a phenothiazine drug and this group is known to produce bronchodilation.

Aitkenhead A and Smith G (2008) *Textbook of Anaesthesia*, 5th edition. Edinburgh: Churchill Livingstone.
Peck T, Hill S, and Williams M (2004) *Pharmacology for Anaesthesia and Intensive Care*, 2nd edition. Cambridge: Cambridge University Press.

27 Hyperglycaemia may be associated with:

a **False** Isoprenaline causes the release of insulin and counteracts any rise in glucose produced by its other beta activity.
b **False** Epidural anaesthesia does not cause any change in blood sugar.
c **False** Thiopental has no effect on blood sugar.
d **False** Ketamine does not affect glucose control.
e **False** Except diethyl ether in the past, none of the inhalational agents produce any elevation of blood sugar.

Aitkenhead A and Smith G (2008) *Textbook of Anaesthesia*, 5th edition. Edinburgh: Churchill Livingstone.
Peck T, Hill S, and Williams M (2004) *Pharmacology for Anaesthesia and Intensive Care*, 2nd edition. Cambridge: Cambridge University Press.

28 Drugs increasing cerebral blood flow include:

a **True** All inhalational agents have a similar effect, some greater than others. Halothane was particularly avoided in neurosurgery.

b **True** Enflurane, in common with the other inhalational agents, causes dose-dependent vasodilation and increases cerebral blood flow. Inhalational agents also abolish autoregulation although sevoflurane has the least effect compared with the other agents.

c **True** Ketamine must therefore be used with caution in hypertension and in those with raised intracranial pressure.

d **False** It has a protective effect on the brain by reducing its oxygen consumption. It is not implicated in any rise in intracranial pressure.

e **False** Thiopental reduces cerebral perfusion pressure and intracranial pressure.

Peck T, Hill S, and Williams M (2004) *Pharmacology for Anaesthesia and Intensive Care*, 2nd edition. Cambridge: Cambridge University Press.

29 Heparin exerts its anticoagulant action by:

a **True** Heparin binds to antithrombin III, increasing its activity by a factor of 1000. The antithrombin–thrombin complex that is formed is inactive, thus preventing conversion of fibrinogen to fibrin.

b **True** Thrombin formation is prevented by inhibiting factor Xa and also by increasing formation of the antithrombin–thrombin complex.

c **True** Heparin inhibits factor Xa, which in turn reduces conversion of prothrombin to thrombin and therefore also reduces conversion of fibrinogen to fibrin.

d **True** Platelet adhesion and aggregation are inhibited at higher doses.

e **True** Heparin aids clot resolution.

Peck T, Hill S, and Williams M (2004) *Pharmacology for Anaesthesia and Intensive Care*, 2nd edition. Cambridge: Cambridge University Press.

30 Anaesthetic drugs that are safe in dystrophia myotonica include:

a **False** Suxamethonium is one of the drugs known to produce myotonic contractions.

b **True** It has been shown to be safe.

c **False** Thiopental (thiopentone) produces severe respiratory depression in these patients and is to be avoided.

d **False** They are sensitive opiates as well and opiate dose needs to be decreased.

e **False** Anticholinesterase injection produces a sudden surge of acetylcholine, which can trigger a myotonic reaction. If muscle relaxation is required, atracurium may be used in small doses, allowing time for the effect of the agent to wear off instead of using neostigmine.

Peck T, Hill S, and Williams M (2004) *Pharmacology for Anaesthesia and Intensive Care*, 2nd edition. Cambridge: Cambridge University Press.

chapter

2

PHYSICS

QUESTIONS

1 Concerning ultrasound:

a Sound waves with a frequency >20 000 Hz are termed ultrasound
b Velocity of sound in air = 330 m/s
c Absorption of ultrasound by tissues generates heat
d For an abdominal scan a frequency of up to 10 MHz is required
e For an ophthalmological investigation a frequency of 2–3.5 MHz is needed

2 Oesophageal Doppler monitoring:

a Is useful in guidance of fluid replacement
b Utilizes a probe with the tip positioned approximately 40 cm from the upper teeth
c Calculates the stroke volume as: flow velocity × ejection time × cross-sectional area of the aorta
d Demonstrates the patient is hypovolaemic when the corrected flow velocity time (FTc) is <0.35 s
e Is a useful guide to cardiac output in the awake patient

3 Regarding logarithms:

a It is the power to which a fixed number (base) must be raised to produce a given number.
b It is used to compress a numerical value
c Two numbers may be multiplied together by adding the logarithms of the numbers.
d The pH of normal blood is given as $-pH = \log(4) + \log(10^{-8})$
e When the pH of blood drops from 7.4 to 7.1 the total amount of acid in the blood is twice as much.

4 Concerning osmolality and osmolarity:

a The osmoles of a solute in 1 litre of solution are expressed as the osmolality (osmol/l of solution)
b Osmolarity is related to the number of particles present in 1 kg of solvent (osmol/l of solvent)
c The tonicity of a substance refers to the effective osmotic pressure relative to plasma
d Osmolarity is more relevant in clinical situations, e.g. in pharmaceutical manufacture of chemical solutions
e Osmometers measure the osmolarity by depression of the freezing point

5 The following SI units denote specific terms:

a	Work (newton)	=	energy/second
b	Energy (joule)	=	force × distance
c	Frequency (Hz)	=	cycles/minute
d	Power (watt)	=	energy/ second
e	Electrical potential (volt)	=	power/current

6 A capacitor:

- a Is made up of two conductors (plates) separated by an insulator
- b Is capable of storing and discharging electricity
- c Is the main component of a defibrillator (external or implanted)
- d Will allow direct current to flow
- e Discharges exponentially therefore discharge = resistance × capacitance

7 A diode:

- a Is a semiconductor
- b Allows bidirectional flow
- c Is made of silicon
- d When connected back to back to another diode, it is called a transistor
- e Is used frequently as a rectifier to allow signals of one polarity to flow but reject signals of the opposite polarity

8 Regarding direct current:

- a When there is a potential difference between two points on a conductor a current will flow
- b Is the mode used in electrical defibrillators
- c A resistor is used in the circuit to reduce the voltage applied to distal components
- d When two resistors are used in series the resistance is given as:

$$\frac{1}{R} = \frac{1}{R_1} + \frac{1}{R_2}$$

- e Work done by the current passing through a resistor is power, i.e. energy/unit time, given as watt.

9 Concerning surgical diathermy:

- a Heat generated by a current passing through a resistor to the tissues is the principle underlying diathermy
- b By increasing the frequency of the alternating current, the electric shock effect is separated from the heating effect
- c Frequency of >1500 kHz is required for coagulation
- d Frequency of >2500 kHz is required for cutting
- e Burns occur if inadvertent contact is made between with some antiseptic solutions and the return plate

10 A silicon strain gauge:

- a Acts as the transducer into which a four-arm bridge is fused
- b Is used in measuring blood pressure
- c Is 10 times more sensitive than ordinary transducers
- d Can be affected by temperature variations
- e Can handle a pressure range of 0–300 mmHg efficiently

11 Regarding scavenging in operating theatres:

- a Anaesthetic agents from floor level are vented as fresh air is pumped in from higher up
- b May involve adsorption of anaesthetic agents
- c Activated charcoal is produced by irradiating charcoal
- d Direct suction attached to the expiratory valve is an efficient option
- e Assisted passive systems route expired gases to a unidirectional exhaust system.

12 Cylinder sizes and capacities:

- a Oxygen is available in four different sizes of cylinder: C, D, E, and F
- b An F size cylinder of oxygen contains 1360 litres
- c Nitrous oxide is available in three cylinder sizes: C, D, and E
- d Air cylinders are G and J size
- e Oxygen and helium mixture (Heliox) cylinders are available in three sizes: D, E, and F

13 To safeguard against delivery of a hypoxic mixture:

- a The oxygen flow meter should be positioned to the right of the flow meter bank
- b The pin-index system should be checked before mounting the cylinder on to the anaesthetic machine
- c A 'tug test' should be performed on the pipeline to check for a firm connection
- d A Bosun whistle, an efficient warning device to indicate oxygen failure, should be connected to every anaesthetic machine
- e The emergency oxygen delivery should be positioned proximal to the flow meters

14 Gas analysis may be performed using the following:

- a Polarography
- b Mass spectrometry
- c Paramagnetism
- d Thermal conductivity
- e Adsorption on to polymers

15 Regarding endotracheal tubes:

- a Of the red rubber variety (Magill tube) used in the past were irritant to the airway because of the mineralized (zinc) rubber
- b That are disposable are made of polyvinyl chloride (PVC)
- c That are armoured are strengthened by wire or nylon
- d Cuff pressure should be maintained at or below 40 cmH_2O to prevent damage to the tracheal mucosa during long-term ventilation
- e The distance from the upper incisor to the manubriosternal junction can be taken as a guide to the length of endotracheal tube required

16 In statistics:

- a The larger the population in the study, the smaller the standard deviation and the greater the reliability
- b Variance is the square root of standard deviation
- c The 'chi-squared test' compares the observed and the expected results thus:

$$\frac{(\text{observed results} - \text{expected})^2}{\text{expected}}$$

  to calculate the significance
- d A 'p' value greater than 0.05 indicates that the results are significant
- e The null hypothesis assumes that the results could not have been produced purely by chance

17 Hot water humidifiers:

- a Should be heated to 60°C to prevent bacterial colonization
- b Are placed above the level of the patient
- c Should have delivery tubing made as short as possible
- d Have a second thermostat as a back-up
- e Reliably ensure the absence of spore-bearing organisms in the water

18 The Aldasorber:

- a Is a passive scavenging system
- b Is a canister containing soda lime and activated charcoal
- c Adsorbs all anaesthetic agents
- d Provides a visual indicator when its contents are exhausted
- e Releases the inhalational agents when heated

19 The Mapleson E breathing circuit:

- a Is used in children weighing up to 30 kg
- b Can be connected easily to the scavenging system
- c Requires gas flow to equal the minute ventilation during spontaneous ventilation
- d May be used for invasive positive pressure ventilation (IPPV) by removing the bag and connecting it to a ventilator
- e Reservoir tubing should be three times the patient's tidal volume

20 Self-inflating bag and masks for resuscitation:

- a Possess a non-rebreathing valve
- b Are only suitable for controlled ventilation
- c Have an inspiratory resistance of 2 cmH_2O
- d Have a reservoir bag for additional oxygen supply
- e Are single use

21 A thermistor:

- a Is a semiconducting element
- b Could be made from oxides of manganese, nickel, cobalt, iron, or zinc
- c Uses the 'Seebeck effect' in measuring temperature
- d Is capable of measuring changes in temperature rapidly
- e Resistance decreases as temperature increases

22 Regarding peripheral nerve stimulators:

- a They use an electrical pulse to depolarize all motor nerve fibres in a peripheral nerve to elicit a response from the muscle
- b A 'train-of-four' technique uses four successive stimuli at one second intervals
- c The sequence of four stimuli may only be repeated every 30 seconds in the train-of-four
- d A two-twitch response on train-of-four monitoring is adequate for most general surgical procedures
- e May be helpful in diagnosing a cholinergic crisis

23 In assessing reversal of muscle relaxants with a peripheral nerve stimulator:

- a Reversal with neostigmine is not possible if there are no twitches seen on a train-of-four
- b Post-tetanic response of increased twitch height is indicative of suitable conditions for reversal
- c Placement over the ulnar nerve correlates well with degree of relaxation of abdominal muscles
- d Double-burst stimulation may be better than train-of-four for guiding the timing of reversal
- e Twitch response followed by sustained tetanic contraction and no post-tetanic potentiation would be indicative of no residual block

24 Breathing circuits:

- a Mapleson A is the most efficient for spontaneous ventilation
- b Mapleson D is the most efficient for controlled ventilation
- c Mapleson D is better than B and C for spontaneous respiration
- d The original Mapleson E (Ayres T piece) required a fresh gas flow rate of approximately three times the minute volume
- e With the Jackson–Rees modification, the function of the Mapleson E circuit is unaffected if gas flow rate equals three times the minute volume

25 Concerning humidification of inspired gases:

- a It is necessary for all intubated patients
- b A heated water bath humidifier is used during long-term ventilation
- c The gas driven heated nebulizers are as effective as ultrasonic nebulizers
- d A heat and moisture exchanger (HME) is adequate for the majority of patients
- e In a patient who is hypothermic (<32°C) HMEs are contraindicated

26 Regarding electrical safety in operating theatres:

- a All interconnected electrical appliances must be connected to the same phase supply called the star point
- b A difference in the current flowing between live and neutral wires is called the leakage current
- c Earth leakage (due to faulty earthing) should not exceed 0.5 mA
- d A surge test is employed to test the integrity of the earth wire, and is called the earth continuity test
- e The resistance between the earth pin and the main earth terminal on the device being tested should not be greater than 1 Ohm

27 Regarding microshock:

- a It is a term applied when cardiac irregularities occur with very small leakage currents during invasive procedures
- b It does not occur until currents of 1 mA are applied
- c Substantially large currents in the order of 10 mA are required to affect atrial function
- d The threshold for shock is also dependent on the frequency of the current which determines the effect
- e The British standard specifies that all equipment in the vicinity of the patient should have a normal leakage current of <10 μA, rising to no more than 50 μA under fault conditions.

28 The Servo-*i* ventilator:

- a Is most suited to intensive care patient use
- b Is only used for adult patients
- c Depends on mains electricity supply to function
- d Can be used to deliver anaesthetic gases in theatre
- e Has a mode for CPAP

29 Regarding waveforms and their display:

- a Fourier was the first to introduce analysis of a waveform
- b A complex waveform contains a fundamental frequency and a series of harmonics
- c A simple wave form is called a sinusoid or simple harmonic waveform
- d The sharper the waveform under examination, the more harmonics will be required to represent it
- e The frequency response of a transducer is vital to enable the device to follow the most rapidly moving parts in a particular waveform

30 The Manley ventilator:

- a Is an example of a gas-driven ventilator
- b Is a minute volume divider
- c Inspiratory to expiratory ratio can be set by altering the gas flow.
- d Is a constant pressure generator during inspiration
- e Cycling from inspiration to expiration is volume cycled

chapter 2

PHYSICS

ANSWERS

1 Concerning ultrasound:

a **True** Above a frequency of 20 000 Hz or 20 kHz, the human ear is unable to register sound and hence it is termed 'ultrasound'. Frequencies used in ultrasound imaging are commonly between 2 MHz and 12 MHz (1 kHz = 1000 Hz; 1 MHz = 1 000 000 Hz).

b **True** Sound travels through different media at different rates and in water it travels at 1480 m/s or approximately four times faster than in air and in bone at 4080 m/s or over 12 times faster.

c **True** As the ultrasound moves through the tissue, some of the signal is lost or attenuated by reflection, scattering, and absorption. The process of absorption is the conversion of sound energy into heat energy in the tissues. As a consequence the surrounding tissues heat up. This is the principle used in the ultrasound treatment of injuries in physiotherapy.

d **False** The frequency of ultrasound selected depends on the depth of tissue penetration required. A higher frequency will provide better quality images but with less tissue penetration and vice versa. A frequency of 3–5 MHz is used for abdominal scanning to achieve a depth of approximately 16 cm.

e **False** Frequencies of 10 MHz can be used in ophthalmological investigations where a depth of only 2.5 cm may be required, but with high resolution.

Sykes M, Vickers M, and Hull C (1991) *Principles of Clinical Measurement*, 3rd revised edition. Oxford: Wiley Blackwell.

2 Oesophageal Doppler:

a **True** The oesophageal Doppler method of cardiac output monitoring involves inserting a probe orally so that the transducer lies adjacent to the descending aorta. An aortic velocity signal is obtained from movement of blood within the aorta, and this is then used, with an estimate of the cross-section of the aorta, to calculate the cardiac output and other parameters such as stroke volume, which can be used as endpoints to resuscitation or fluid replacement.

b **True** This distance from the upper incisors corresponds roughly to the mid-thoracic level of the descending aorta, which is required for the measurements.

c **True** When the aortic velocity signal is obtained, this is used in conjunction with the cross-sectional area of the aorta (estimated from the patient's age, height, and weight) to calculate the stroke volume.

d **True** The base of the waveform is used as a measure of preload. FTc is the systolic flow time in seconds, corrected for the heart rate. When the FTc is low, it can indicate that the preload is low (i.e. hypovolaemia) or that the afterload is high.

e **False** The oesophageal Doppler probes are approximately 6 mm in diameter and are semi-rigid, which means that their use is limited to the intubated and sedated patient. A more flexible probe suitable use in awake patients is being introduced.

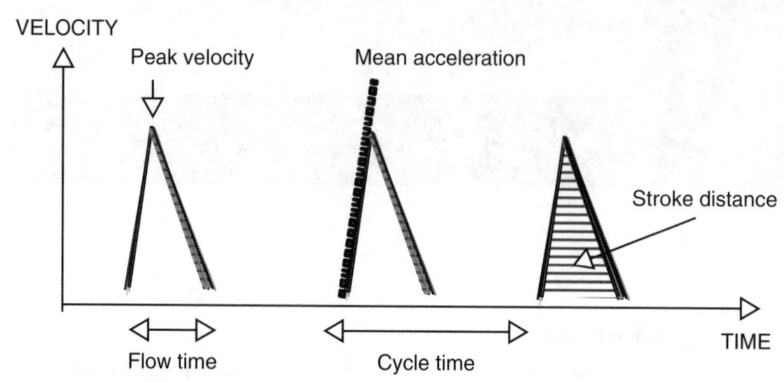

Figure 2.4 Doppler velocity–time waveform.

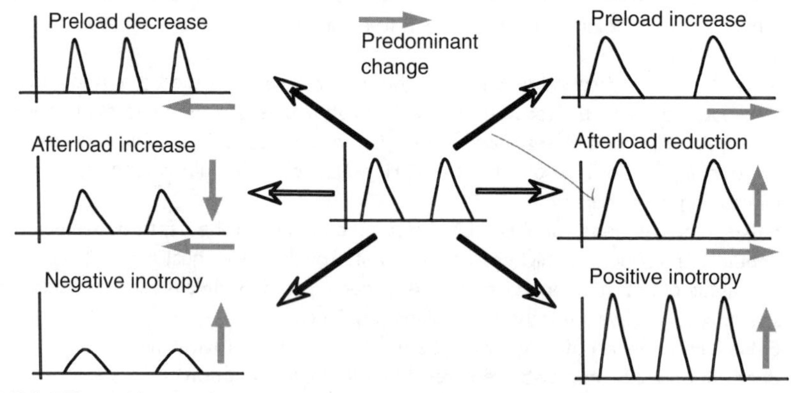

Figure 2.5 Effect of haemodynamic changes on Doppler velocity–time waveform shape.
Reproduced from Singer M and Webb A (2006) *Oxford Handbook of Critical Care*, 2nd edition. New York: Oxford University Press.

Singer M and Webb A (2006) *Oxford Handbook of Critical Care*, 2nd edition. New York: Oxford University Press.
Sykes M, Vickers M, and Hull C (1991) *Principles of Clinical Measurement*, 3rd revised edition. Wiley Blackwell.

3 Regarding logarithms:

a **True** For example $10^5 = 100\ 000$, i.e. 10 multiplied by itself five times. The figure 5 is termed the index or exponent and indicates that 10 has to be raised to the power of 5. The 5 may be referred to as the logarithm of 100 000 to the base 10, and expressed as $\log_{10}(100\ 000) = 5$.

b **True** For example the normal hydrogen ion concentration is 0.00 000 004 g/l or 4 parts out of 100 000 000 *or* 4×10^{-8} g/l.
Since $pH = -\log_{10}[H^+]$, it can be rewritten as $-pH = \log(4) + \log(10^{-8})$ *or* $= 0.6 - 8 = -7.4$ *or* pH=7.4.

c **True** By simply adding two logarithms of numbers their value can be ascertained using the antilog tables.

d **True** As in the derivation in part b, this is another way of representing pH 7.4.

e **True** At normal pH of 7.4 the H^+ ion concentration is 39.8 nmol/l and at a pH of 7.1 the concentration is 79.4 mmol/l.

Sykes M, Vickers M, and Hull C (1991) *Principles of Clinical Measurement*, 3rd revised edition. Wiley Blackwell.

4 Regarding osmolality and osmolarity:

a **False** Osmolality is the number of osmoles dissolved in 1 kg of solvent. The unit is mmol/kg. Osmoles are calculated from the molecular weight of a substance divided by the number of free-moving particles liberated in solution.

b **False** Osmolarity is the number of osmoles present in 1 litre of solution. The unit is mmol/l.

c **True** If a substance is hypotonic, it has less osmotic pressure relative to the plasma, isotonic is equal, and a hypertonic solution exerts more osmotic pressure than the plasma.

d **True** In all pharmacological preparations, it is more common to take osmolarity as the standard with which a solution is prepared.

e **True** Osmometers are used to measure the osmolality of urine or plasma. It works on the principle of depression of the freezing point of a solution, the depression of the freezing point being directly proportional to the osmolality. When 1 mol of a substance is added to 1 kg of water, it depresses the freezing point by 1.86°C. For example, if the osmolality of the plasma increases, the freezing point of the water in the plasma will decrease and this is detected by the osmometer.

Davis P and Kenny G (2002) *Basic Physics and Measurement in Anaesthesia*, 5th edition. Boston, MA: Butterworth-Heinemann.

5 The following SI units denote specific terms:

a **False** Work is done or energy is used when the point of application of a force moves in the direction of the force. The SI unit of energy is the joule. The newton is a measure of force and has the unit $kg.m/s^2$.

b **True** The joule (J) is a measure of energy or work. It equates to force × distance and has the unit Nm.

c **False** Frequency has the unit hertz (Hz), and 1 Hz has a frequency of 1 cycle/s.

d **True** Power is equivalent to the rate of energy expenditure. It is measured in watts (W). 1 W = 1 J/s.

e **True** Electrical potential is measured in volts (V) and 1 V is the difference in potential between two points carrying a current of 1 ampere (A) when the power dissipated between these points is 1 W. It is also expressed as V = W/A.

Davis P and Kenny G (2002) *Basic Physics and Measurement in Anaesthesia*, 5th edition. Boston, MA: Butterworth-Heinemann.

6 A capacitor:

a **True** A capacitor is a device that stores electrical charge. When connected to a source of electricity the current will flow into the capacitor and is stored as an electric charge until it is discharged by the operator.
b **True** It is the function of the capacitor to store and discharge electricity.
c **True** Energy stored in the capacitor is discharged as a current pulse (5–10 ms) causing synchronous contraction of the heart after which a refractory period and normal rhythm may follow.
d **False** The capacitor will not allow flow of direct current. It acts as a low frequency filter, retarding the flow of low frequency or direct current. The capacitor will, however, allow alternating current to pass as it is continuously being charged and discharged, allowing current to flow.
e **True** The rate of decay of the current is exponential when passing through the capacitor.

Davis P and Kenny G (2002) *Basic Physics and Measurement in Anaesthesia*, 5th edition. Boston, MA: Butterworth-Heinemann.

7 A diode:

a **True** A diode is a semiconductor.
b **False** Resistors, capacitors, and inductors can be connected either way round as the current will pass equally well in both directions. A diode is a unidirectional device that allows current to flow in only one direction.
c **True** They are mostly made from silicon, although germanium and selenium have been used.
d **True** The current flowing in one diode can bring about large changes in the current flowing in the second diode, and thus amplification of the signal Is obtained. Transistors have almost entirely replaced valves in electronic circuitry.
e **True** Diodes are frequently used for this purpose, which will allow signals of one polarity to flow but reject signals of the opposite polarity; they are analogous to a unidirectional valve.

Sykes M, Vickers M, and Hull C (1991) *Principles of Clinical Measurement*, 3rd revised edition. Wiley Blackwell.

8 Regarding direct current:

a **True** It is a unidirectional flow of current, which in the past was called 'galvanic current'. I = E/R where I = current, E= potential difference, and R = resistance.
b **True** Alternating current is not capable of an adequate build-up of charge for defibrillation in the required time. Direct current is used as it is more effective and is less damaging than alternating current.
c **True** They may also be used to separate components by a fixed voltage.
d **False** When connected in series the resistance is the sum of the two resistors. When they are connected in *parallel*, it is the reciprocal of the two.
e **True** Power in watts (W) is the rate of energy expenditure. One watt is equal to one joule per second (1 W = 1 J/s).

Davis P and Kenny G (2002) *Basic Physics and Measurement in Anaesthesia*, 5th edition. Boston, MA: Butterworth-Heinemann.

9 Concerning surgical diathermy:

a **True** When an electric current is passed through a resistor heating occurs. This is a similar principle to an electric fire.

b **True** Diathermy is made safe by the use of high frequency current. The highest risk of shocks and arrhythmias occur at 50 Hz, which is the mains frequency in the UK. The operating frequency of the surgical diathermy machine current is in the region of 0.5–1 MHz, thus greatly reducing the risk of adverse effects.

c **False** A frequency of 400 kHz is adequate for coagulation. Coagulation uses a lower frequency current and a pulsed sine wave pattern.

d **False** A frequency of 1500 kHz is required for cutting. Cutting uses a higher frequency current and a continuous sine wave pattern.

e **True** Burns may be caused by mercurial salts found in some antiseptic solutions. Another major cause of burns is ignition of pools of spirit-based skin preparation fluids, resulting in contact or flash burns.

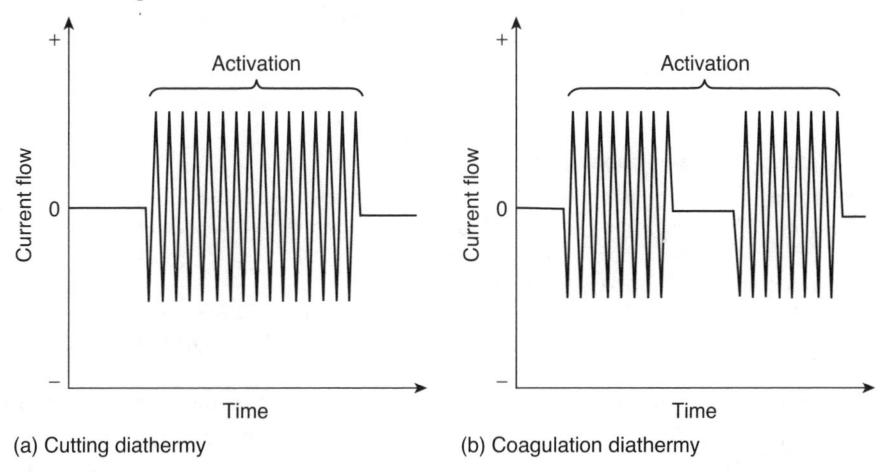

Figure 2.6 Cutting and coagulation diathermy.
Reproduced with kind permission from Cross M and Plunkett E (2008) *Physics, Pharmacology and Physiology for Anaesthetists*. Cambridge: Cambridge University Press.

Cross M and Plunkett E (2008) *Physics, Pharmacology and Physiology for Anaesthetists*. Cambridge: Cambridge University Press.
Davis P and Kenny G (2002) *Basic Physics and Measurement in Anaesthesia*, 5th edition. Boston, MA: Butterworth-Heinemann.

10 A silicon strain gauge:

a **True** A silicon strain gauge is used to form one of the four arms of the balanced Wheatstone bridge circuit. A change in pressure causes the resistance of the strain gauge to alter which registers a current.

b **True** These can be made very small and have been incorporated in the tip of cardiac catheters as well as being employed in invasive arterial monitoring.

c **True** Silicon strain gauges are more sensitive than wire strain gauge elements.

d **True** They can exhibit a thermal drift compared to other types of transducers. The current products however, seem to be more stable under different temperatures.

e **True** Thus they are suitable for invasive monitoring and diagnostics.

Scurr C, Feldman S, and Soni N (1990) *Scientific Foundations of Anaesthesia*, 4th edition. Oxford: Butterworth-Heinemann.

11 Regarding scavenging in operating theatres:

a **True** The frequent and rapid changing of the circulating air (15–20 times per hour) is one of the most important factors in reducing theatre pollution. This non-recirculating ventilation system gives the maximum benefit.

b **True** The Cardiff Aldasorber is a canister containing activated charcoal for adsorption of inhalational agents. Nitrous oxide is not removed and the capacity is limited necessitating frequent changes.

c **False** When charcoal is heated under anaerobic conditions it becomes more porous and thereby the surface area for adsorption is increased. The term 'activated' refers to this process and has nothing to with radiation.

d **False** Applying direct suction to the expiratory valve has the risk of sucking out the anaesthetic gases and oxygen from the breathing circuit.

e **False** The scavenging system employed in most theatres is an active system where a vacuum is created by providing suction beyond a reservoir system where the expired gases are routed from the patient end. The removal from the reservoir is active and the gases are then vented into the atmosphere.

Al-Shaikh B and Stacey S (2006) *Essentials of Anaesthetic Equipment*, 3rd edition. Edinburgh: Churchill Livingstone.

12 Cylinder sizes and capacities:

a **False** Oxygen cylinders for medical use come in six sizes: C, D, E, F, G, and J.

b **True** The sizes G and J contain 3400 and 6800 litres, respectively, and can be used in a central cylinder supply manifold in hospitals too small to require a vacuum insulated evaporator (VIE) for oxygen storage.

c **False** Nitrous oxide cylinders are available in five sizes: C, D, E, F, and G.

d **True** These compressed air cylinders are frequently used in the orthopaedic theatres if pipeline air supply is not available.

e **True** D, E, and F cylinders contain 300, 600, and 1200 litres of this mixture, respectively.

Al-Shaikh B and Stacey S (2006) *Essentials of Anaesthetic Equipment*, 3rd edition. Edinburgh: Churchill Livingstone.

13 To safeguard against delivery of a hypoxic mixture:

a **True** Although this seems an obvious answer, the anaesthetic machines in the UK have the oxygen flow meter on the left side of the bank.

b **True** With the pin-index system it is almost impossible to fix the cylinders to the wrong position on the machine.

c **True** The 'tug test' is a routine test that should be performed as part of the checks of the anaesthetic machine before use.

d **False** The Bosun warning device relied on a battery power supply for a warning light and only worked when nitrous oxide was connected. It also provided a warning whistle. The present day devices depend only on the pressure of oxygen and no additional power supply such as a battery. As an additional safety feature they will also cut off all the anaesthetic gases and open the circuit to atmospheric air when the oxygen supply fails and they cannot be switched off.

e **False** The emergency oxygen should bypass all the flow meters and vaporizers, and supply oxygen directly to the patient.

Aitkenhead A and Smith G (2008) *Textbook of Anaesthesia*, 5th edition. Edinburgh: Churchill Livingstone.
Al-Shaikh B and Stacey S (2006) *Essentials of Anaesthetic Equipment*, 3rd edition. Edinburgh: Churchill Livingstone.

14 Gas analysis may be performed using the following:

a **True** Oxygen and nitrous oxide can be analysed with this method.

b **True** Mass spectrometers are capable of separating the components of complex gas mixtures according to their mass and charge.

c **True** Only two gases, oxygen and nitric oxide, are attracted by a magnetic field, i.e. they are paramagnetic.

d **True** A gas with high thermal conductivity conducts heat more readily than the one with low conductivity. This principle is used in katharometers. The degree of cooling of a heated wire is dependent on the temperature of the gas, the rate of gas flow, and the thermal conductivity of the gas.

e **True** Adsorption of inhalational agents onto silicone bands causes the bands to elongate, and the degree of relaxation is recorded. This property of adsorption onto polymers was used in the 'Narko test' in the past.

Sykes M, Vickers M, and Hull C (1991) *Principles of Clinical Measurement*, 3rd revised edition. Wiley Blackwell.

15 Regarding endotracheal tubes:

a **True** Red rubber tubes were suitable for short-term intubation only due to the nature of the reinforced rubber, which can cause severe laryngeal irritation leading to oedema. One of the minerals contained in the mixture forming the red rubber is believed to be zinc, which is responsible for the local irritation. The red rubber tube was also expensive to use and would deteriorate on repeated sterilization.

b **True** Since the advent of PVC tubes the management of patients on artificial ventilators has become safer, and patients can now be intubated for longer periods because of the inert nature of PVC.

c **True** Endotracheal tubes can be reinforced by the addition of a spiral of either nylon or metal wire in their wall, and are used when kinking of the endotracheal tube is anticipated, for example in neurosurgery or cases involving a shared airway such as in maxillofacial surgery.

d **True** Although it is debated periodically, there is no unanimous view on what the safe pressure in a tracheal tube cuff should be. Some argue that it should be less than 30 cmH_2O, but a compromise figure of 40 cmH_2O is accepted by most.

e **True** The distance from the upper incisor to the carina is approximately 24 cm. If a tube is held against side of the patient's face and the distance noted, the tracheal tube should be positioned a minimum of 2–3 cm from the carina.

Aitkenhead A and Smith G. (2008) *Textbook of Anaesthesia*, 5th edition. Edinburgh: Churchill Livingstone.

16 In statistics:

a **True** The larger the population, the less is the element of chance occurrence.

b **False** Standard deviation is the square root of variance. Variance is the sum of squares of the differences divided by the degrees of freedom.

c **True** This is one of the basic tests of significance.

d **False** A 'p' value smaller than 0.05 will be significant, i.e. 0.01 has greater significance than 0.05.

e **False** The null hypothesis assumes that there is no difference between the groups being studied.

Scurr C, Feldman S, and Soni N (1990) *Scientific Foundations of Anaesthesia*, 4th edition. Oxford: Butterworth-Heinemann.

17 Hot water humidifiers:

a **True** Most forms of bacteria are destroyed at this temperature.

b **False** They should always be placed below the level of patient to avoid hot water entering the patient's airway and causing scalding.

c **True** Short lengths of tubing prevent excessive condensation of water along the circuit.

d **True** A thermostat controls the temperature of the water and it is essential to have a back-up to avoid accidentally high temperatures.

e **False** Spore-bearing organisms are not destroyed at the temperatures at which humidifiers operate.

Al-Shaikh B and Stacey S (2006) *Essentials of Anaesthetic Equipment*, 3rd edition. Edinburgh: Churchill Livingstone.

18 The Aldasorber:

a **True** It was one of the earliest scavenging devices used in theatres.

b **False** It contains activated charcoal only.

c **False** Only halogenated anaesthetic agents are adsorbed onto the charcoal, when expired gases are directed into the canister. It cannot adsorb nitrous oxide.

d **False** The increasing weight of the canister is the only way of determining that it is exhausted.

e **True** There is a danger of theatre pollution if the canister is not disposed of promptly.

Al-Shaikh B and Stacey S (2006) *Essentials of Anaesthetic Equipment*, 3rd edition. Edinburgh: Churchill Livingstone.

19 The Mapleson E breathing system:

a **True** It can be used for children weighing up to 25–30 kg.

b **False** It is not easy to efficiently scavenge expired gases from the Mapleson E system unless it is modified to a Mapleson F circuit by the addition of an adjustable pressure limiting (APL) valve and a closed-ended reservoir bag.

c **False** A fresh gas flow of 2.5–3 times the minute volume is required to prevent rebreathing.

d **True** A ventilator such as a Penlon Nuffield 200 may be used for IPPV.

e **False** The volume of the reservoir tubing should be equal to the patient's tidal volume. If the tubing is too small, air will be entrained and if it is too large, rebreathing will occur.

Al-Shaikh B and Stacey S (2006) *Essentials of Anaesthetic Equipment*, 3rd edition. Edinburgh: Churchill Livingstone.

20 Self-inflating bag and masks for resuscitation:

a **True** A non-rebreathing Ambu® valve is an essential component of the system.

b **False** They can be used for both spontaneous and controlled ventilation.

c **False** The Ambu® valve provides only a small resistance to flow. At a gas flow rate of 25 l/min the inspiratory resistance is just 0.4 cmH_2O.

d **True** The addition of a reservoir bag allows a higher fraction of inspired oxygen (FiO_2) to be delivered to the patient.

e **True** Both adult and paediatric single-use designs are in common use.

Al-Shaikh B and Stacey S (2006) *Essentials of Anaesthetic Equipment*, 3rd edition. Edinburgh: Churchill Livingstone.

21 A thermistor:

a **True** A thermistor is a semiconductor that possesses a negative temperature coefficient of resistance. The beads of heavy metal oxide that the thermistor is composed of have small thermal capacities and rapid response times.

b **True** They are composed of small beads of heavy metal oxides (e.g. manganese, nickel, zinc, cobalt, and iron).

c **False** The 'Seebeck effect' is utilized in the thermocouple, where the difference in the potential difference between a reference electrode that is kept at a steady temperature and the measuring electrode denotes the temperature.

d **True** They have a small thermal capacity and can respond rapidly to changes in temperature—in as little as 0.2 seconds.

e **True** In contrast to the resistance wire where resistance increases as the temperature increases, the resistance of certain semiconductor metals decreases as temperature increases. This is a non-linear relationship but can be converted to a linear relationship for ease of interpretation.

Pinnock C, Lin T, and Smith T (2002) *Fundamentals of Anaesthesia*, 2nd edition. New York: Cambridge University Press.

22 Regarding peripheral nerve stimulators:

a **True** They exhaust the acetylcholine at all nerve terminals to produce maximum depolarization at the muscle receptors (supramaximal stimulation).

b **False** The train-of-four technique uses four stimuli at 0.5 second intervals. The train-of-four ratio is the amplitude of the fourth twitch divided by the amplitude of the first twitch given in a ratio T4:T1.

c **False** It may be repeated every 10–15 seconds.

d **True** A two-twitch response on train-of-four monitoring indicates approximately 80% blockade of neuromuscular junction receptors and is suitable for most general surgical procedures for maintenance.

e **True** It will demonstrate the presence of a dense block.

Aitkenhead A and Smith G. (2008) *Textbook of Anaesthesia*, 5th edition. Edinburgh: Churchill Livingstone.

23 In assessing reversal of muscle relaxants with a peripheral nerve stimulator:

a **True** A train-of-four count of greater than three twitches is required before attempting reversal of neuromuscular blockade with neostigmine. This is especially the case with long-acting agents. Reversal of rocuronium with sugammadex, however, does not require any twitches on train-of-four monitoring.

b **True** The post-tetanic count is used when the block is intense and no twitches are seen on train-of-four. The tetanic stimulus releases acetylcholine, so that on repeated train-of-four stimulation, a response is seen. The pattern of the response can be interpreted, depending on the agent used, as to the likelihood of return of train-of-four twitches and therefore the possibility of reversal.

c **False** The response of the orbicularis oculi seems to correlate better with abdominal muscle relaxation as this is a central muscle and more resistant to blockade like the diaphragm. The peripheral muscles are more sensitive and may not adequately reflect the degree of block required at a given time.

d **True** The fade in a train-of-four can be difficult to detect especially by comparing the middle two twitches with the first and the last. Double-burst stimulation consists of two sets of twitches separated by a brief interval to improve perception of fade.

e **True** In the investigation of prolonged recovery from anaesthesia, the peripheral nerve stimulator can be used to rule out residual neuromuscular blockade as a cause.

Aitkenhead A and Smith G. (2008) *Textbook of Anaesthesia*, 5th edition. Edinburgh: Churchill Livingstone.

24 Breathing circuits:

a **True** Mapleson 'A' or the Magill's circuit requires a flow rate equal to the alveolar ventilation to prevent rebreathing. When used for controlled ventilation it requires twice the minute ventilation.

b **True** During controlled ventilation all the fresh gas input is delivered to the patient. It is less efficient for spontaneous ventilation.

c **True** More rebreathing occurs with B and C systems.

d **True** Although the flow rate can be reduced to 2–2.5 times the minute volume when the overall expiratory rate is slow during spontaneous respiration, it has to be three times the minute volume during controlled ventilation.

e **True** To prevent rebreathing the expiratory limb should have an internal volume greater than the patient's tidal volume, and hence the flow rate should be three times the minute volume.

Scurr C, Feldman S, and Soni N (1990) *Scientific Foundations of Anaesthesia*, 4th edition. Oxford: Butterworth-Heinemann.

25 Concerning humidification of inspired gases:

a **True** The nasal passages provide approximately 28 mg water per litre of air during normal respiration. This pathway is lost when the patient has been intubated. The patient must therefore receive humidification by other means to prevent complications.

b **True** The heated water will not only humidify, but will assist in preventing cooling of the respiratory tract and is important for efficient functioning of the respiratory cilia. The warmed water will also discourage growth of microorganisms.

c **True** These nebulizers produce droplet sizes between 5 and 20 microns, but they are satisfactory for the majority of cases.

d **True** These passive devices are simple and cost-effective and contribute only minimally to dead space. Expired air condenses on to the device and humidifies the inspired air, along with preservation of heat. Efficiency is up to 90% and they are suitable for most patients, the exceptions being those with copious secretions and requiring long-term ventilation.

e **True** At 32°C patients require more active methods of humidification. HME effectiveness has been shown to be greatly reduced in hypothermic post-cardiac arrest patients on ventilators.

Scurr C, Feldman S, and Soni N (1990) *Scientific Foundations of Anaesthesia*, 4th edition. Oxford: Butterworth-Heinemann.

26 Regarding electrical safety in operating theatres:

a **True** Electrical power usually arrives on the hospital site as a three-phase, 11 000 V supply. This supply is transformed down to three 240 V supplies by a local transformer. For interconnected electrical devices to perform satisfactorily they should all be connected to a single phase supply.

b **True** A leakage current could be also due to faulty insulation between the device and its metal casing, which is not suitably earthed.

c **True** Any device that has a leakage current greater than 0.5 mA should not be used until corrected.

d **True** While testing for earth leakage, a badly frayed earth wire may give a satisfactory reading. When a 'surge test' is applied a 25 A current is passed through the earth pathway for at least five seconds. If any part of the pathway is limited to one or two strands, the strands will rapidly overheat and blow like a 'fuse'.

e **False** The resistance between the earth pin and the main earth terminal on the device should not be greater than 0.1 Ohm.

Sykes M, Vickers M, and Hull C (1991) *Principles of Clinical Measurement*, 3rd revised edition. Wiley Blackwell.

27 Microshock:

a **True** Very small alternating currents when applied to the ventricles can induce arrhythmias.

b **False** Due to the high current density, as little as 100 μA is sufficient to cause ventricular fibrillation when delivered directly to the heart.

c **False** The current required to affect atrial function is several times that of the one affecting ventricles, but not as high as 10 mA.

d **True** The threshold for arrhythmias is proportional to the surface area and the time for which the current is passed. It is also dependent on the frequency and it has been shown that 50 Hz is almost the lethal frequency, this corresponds to the frequency of UK mains supply making electrical safety even more crucial.

e **True** Considering the above it is logical to assume that a leakage current of 100 μA should never be reached during invasive procedures.

Sykes M, Vickers M, and Hull C (1991) *Principles of Clinical Measurement*, 3rd revised edition. Wiley Blackwell.

28 The Servo-*i* ventilator:

a **True** It is a versatile intensive care ventilator with many different modes of ventilation.

b **False** It is used in both adult and paediatric patients.

c **False** It can be used with a 12 V battery for patient transport.

d **False** It is not designed for use with inhalational agents but can be used in theatre if total intravenous anaesthesia (TIVA) is employed.

e **True** Among its many modes of ventilation, continuous positive airway pressure (CPAP) can be applied as a means of weaning a patient from the ventilator.

Al-Shaikh B and Stacey S (2006) *Essentials of Anaesthetic Equipment*, 3rd edition. Edinburgh: Churchill Livingstone.

29 Regarding waveforms and their display:

a **True** However complex a waveform may appear, it can always be analysed as being the sum of series of much simpler wave forms.

b **True** Any complex waveform will consist of sine waves of different frequencies, the slowest (fundamental) frequency and harmonics of the fundamental frequency.

c **True** Several simple waveforms make a complex waveform.

d **True** A sharper waveform will require more harmonics to represent it.

e **True** For an arterial waveform, a 12 Hz frequency response is required, but to record maximum rate and rise of left ventricular pressure the system should be able to respond accurately to a frequency of 30 Hz or higher.

Scurr C, Feldman S, and Soni N (1990) *Scientific Foundations of Anaesthesia*, 4th edition. Oxford: Butterworth-Heinemann.

30 The Manley ventilator:

a **True** It was the first gas-driven ventilator to be used in the operating theatre.

b **True** The Manley ventilator is a minute volume divider or a time cycled pressure generator. All of the fresh gas flow (minute volume) is delivered to the patient divided into preset tidal volumes.

c **False** The tidal volume can be adjusted by the moving the adjustable stop higher or lower, thereby decreasing or increasing the tidal volume. This will affect the inspiratory to expiratory ratio.

d **True** The weight on top of the horizontal beam connected to the bellows is what determines the pressure. Since the weight is constant, the pressure generated will remain constant throughout inspiration.

e **False** Cycling from inspiration to expiration occurs when the storage bellows begin to fill the main bellows with fresh gas. It is time cycled.

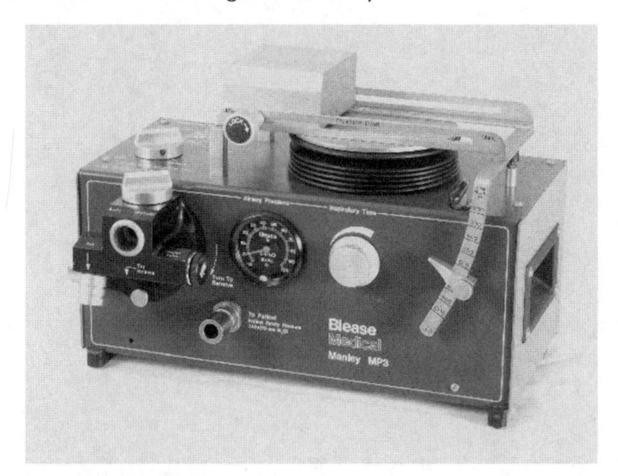

Figure 2.7 The Manley MP3 ventilator.
Reproduced with kind permission from Al-Shaikh B and Stacey S (2006) *Essentials of Anaesthetic Equipment*, 3rd edition. Edinburgh: Churchill Livingstone.

Al-Shaikh B and Stacey S (2006) *Essentials of Anaesthetic Equipment*, 3rd edition. Edinburgh: Churchill Livingstone.

chapter 2 PHYSIOLOGY

QUESTIONS

1 Hypoventilation may result in:

a Hypoxia if the patient breathes air
b Increased plasma bicarbonate
c Decreased pH
d Increased physiological dead space
e Hypercarbia in certain patients receiving supplemental oxygen

2 The cough reflex

a Is mediated through the glossopharyngeal nerves
b Afferent impulses are transmitted to the hypothalamus
c A rapid intake of air in excess of 3 litres precedes the cough
d Intrapulmonary pressure rises to 100 mmHg or more
e Expelled air may reach velocities of 75–100 miles/h

3 Peripheral vascular resistance:

a Is controlled mainly by the cutaneous vessels
b Is a measure of the afterload
c Is decreased with low-dose adrenaline (epinephrine) infusion
d Is increased with low-dose dopamine infusion
e When multiplied by the cardiac output gives the mean blood pressure

4 The following are produced during the synthesis or metabolism of catecholamines:

a Dihydroxyphenylalanine (DOPA)
b 5-hydroxy indole acetic acid
c Beta imidazole ethylamine
d Pipecolyl xylidine
e 3-methoxy 4-hydroxy mandelic acid

5 Neuromuscular block may exist:

a In the presence of hypermagnesaemia
b In botulism
c In association with hyperphosphataemia
d If post-tetanic facilitation is absent after administration of edrophonium
e If both fast (tetanic) and slow (twitch) rates of nerve stimulation are well sustained

6 Compensatory mechanisms during acclimatization to high altitude include:

a Respiratory alkalosis
b Renal conservation of bicarbonate
c Increased erythropoietin secretion
d Increased 2,3-DPG in red cells
e Active transport of H^+ ions into the cerebrospinal fluid (CSF)

7 Breakdown of haemoglobin involves:

a Oxidative cleavage of the porphyrin ring
b Formation of bile pigments
c Recycling of iron from the haem moiety
d Formation of urobilin
e Production of carboxyhaemoglobin

8 Factors increasing the calibre of peripheral blood vessels include:

a Hypothermia
b Hypoxia
c Increased pH
d Serotonin
e Hypercarbia

9 Concerning carbohydrate metabolism:

a All the stages in the metabolic process are insulin dependent
b 28 moles of adenosine triphosphate (ATP) are produced during aerobic glycolysis
c Gluconeogenesis refers to glucose production from amino acids
d The process of glucose conversion to pyruvic acid is known as glycogenolysis
e Usually 30–40% of ingested glucose is converted to fat

10 The tracts in the spinal cord serve the following functions:

a Lateral spinothalamic tract carries touch sensations
b Posterior columns carry touch and proprioception
c Anterior spinothalamic tract carries pain sensation
d Pain fibres are carried by the fasciculus gracilis in the posterior column
e The pyramidal tract (also known as the lateral cerebrospinal tract) is the crossed motor tract descending from the cerebral cortex

11 The following are cholinergic:

a Sympathetic preganglionic fibres
b Splanchnic fibres to the adrenal medulla
c Nerve supply to sweat glands
d Postganglionic sympathetic fibres
e Contractile supply to detrusor muscles

12 The transmission of nerve impulses is:

- a Faster in larger myelinated fibres
- b Affected by hypokalaemia
- c Dependent on the strength and duration of the stimulating current
- d Dependent on metabolism
- e Always unidirectional

13 Cerebral blood flow:

- a Is normally around 1200 ml/min at rest
- b Is increased during mental activity
- c To the grey matter is greater in comparison with the white matter
- d Is not affected significantly by vasomotor reflexes
- e Is increased significantly when the body is accelerated upwards (positive 'G') and results in a 'red out'

14 Haemoglobin:

- a Has a molecular weight of 64 000 daltons
- b Has more affinity for carbon monoxide than oxygen
- c Has alpha and delta chains in the fetus and alpha and beta chains in adults
- d Has a combination of HbS and HbC in sickle cell disease
- e Can take up a further 0.0225 ml of O_2 per 100 ml plasma per kPa increase in PO_2

15 Concerning renal function:

- a Approximately 180 litres of fluid are filtered through the glomeruli each day
- b Water is actively reabsorbed in the proximal tubules
- c Osmolality of the urine is a more sensitive indicator of renal function than its specific gravity
- d Approximately 100 mg/min of glucose is filtered through the glomerulus
- e The clearance of a substance cannot exceed the glomerular filtration rate

16 Concerning the adrenal gland:

- a The medulla is supplied by preganglionic sympathetic fibres that release acetylcholine
- b Normal cortisol secretion is 20 mg/day
- c Normal aldosterone secretion is 2.5 mg/day
- d Metyrapone is a drug that is used to test primary adrenocortical insufficiency
- e Androgens secreted by the adrenal gland are equally effective as testosterone produced by the testes.

17 In nerve muscle physiology:

- a Chronaxie is the shortest time interval during which the weakest current passed will elicit a response
- b Gamma efferent fibres directly control muscle contraction
- c The resting membrane potential in a nerve is –70 mV
- d 35 mV potential is produced during an action potential
- e During the absolute refractory period if a second stimulus of sufficient strength is applied, a response can be elicited

18 Hypercarbia:

- a Decreases blood bicarbonate levels
- b Can exist in the presence of normal PO_2
- c Sensitizes the myocardium to circulating catecholamines
- d Increases cerebral blood flow
- e Increases blood pH

19 Concerning renal physiology:

- a The filtration fraction is the ratio of glomerular filtration rate (GFR) to the renal plasma flow (RPF)
- b Normal GFR in an adult is 125 ml/min
- c The amount of creatinine excreted is approximately equal to the amount filtered
- d Effective filtration pressure at the glomerulus is 15 mmHg (2 kPa)
- e Carbonic anhydrase is essential for hydrogen ion secretion at the proximal and distal tubules.

20 The following are normal values in the cardiovascular system:

- a Left atrial pressure of 5 mmHg
- b Peak right ventricular pressure of 25 mmHg
- c End-diastolic ventricular blood volume of 50 ml
- d PR interval of 0.2 seconds on an electrocardiogram (ECG)
- e Ventricular diastole lasting 0.5 seconds

21 Coronary blood flow:

- a Is dependent on the mean aortic pressure
- b Is maximal in the subendocardial portion of the myocardium during the QRS complex of the ECG
- c Is increased by sympathetic stimulation
- d Is increased by hypoxia
- e Is normally around 250 ml/min at rest

22 Concerning 2,3-diphosphoglycerate (2,3-DPG):

- a Increased levels increase the P50
- b Levels are increased in thyrotoxicosis
- c Levels are decreased in anaemia
- d Levels are increased by exercise
- e It is better preserved in SAGM blood than in the CPD mixture

23 In a patient with obstructive airways disease:

- a Lung compliance is decreased
- b Forced vital capacity (FVC) is decreased
- c Forced expiratory volume in one second (FEV_1) is decreased
- d Maximal voluntary ventilation is reduced
- e Peak expiratory flow rate (PEFR) is decreased

24 Plasma proteins:

- a Normal levels are 60–80 g/l
- b Exert an osmotic pressure of 25 mmHg
- c Are responsible for 30% of the buffering capacity of the blood
- d Are not filtered by the glomeruli
- e Are involved in the transport of hormones, e.g. thyroid hormones and adrenocorticoids

25 In the coagulation system:

- a Platelets are the main source of thromboplastin
- b Serotonin and adenosine diphosphate (ADP) are released to attract platelets to form a plug whenever capillary endothelium is disrupted
- c Plasmin converts fibrinogen to fibrin
- d Factor XI is essential for both the intrinsic and extrinsic pathways of coagulation
- e Factor X deficiency causes haemophilia

26 Regarding temperature regulation:

- a The thermoregulatory centre is mainly situated in the anterior hypothalamus
- b Blood temperature is the most sensitive stimulus to the thermoregulatory centre
- c Core temperature is generally 0.5–1.0°C higher than the oral temperature
- d There is a diurnal fluctuation of temperature in normal individuals
- e Thyroid-stimulating hormone (TSH) secretion is depressed at high body temperatures

27 The pupillary light reflex:

- a Is mediated by the trochlear nerve
- b Is evidenced by constriction of both pupils when light is shone on one eye in the normal individual
- c Is absent in the Argyll Robertson pupil
- d Relay occurs near the mid-brain at the Edinger–Westphal nucleus
- e Long ciliary nerves carry the impulse to the pupillary muscle

28 Among the cranial nerves:

- a The abducens nerve has the longest intracranial course
- b The oculomotor nerve supplies the superior rectus muscle
- c The ophthalmic division of the trigeminal nerve forms the afferent for the oculo-cardiac reflex
- d The glossopharyngeal nerve supplies the anterior surface of the epiglottis
- e The accessory nerve is a purely motor nerve

29 Concerning cardiac output:

- a It can be increased from 5 to 25 l/min during exercise
- b The stroke volume at rest is approximately 40 ml in an adult
- c Athletes are able to exceed a cardiac output of 35 l/min
- d The Fick principle is used for measuring the cardiac output
- e Heart transplant recipients cannot raise their cardiac output in response to exercise

30 In control of respiration:

a 'Apneustic respiration' is a feature after transection at the inferior level of the pons

b The respiratory centre is more sensitive to changes in carbon dioxide levels than oxygen levels

c The 'Hering Breuer reflex' assists in controlling the respiratory rate

d Reflexes mediated by the carotid and aortic bodies stimulate respiration in anaemia

e Kussmaul respiration is seen in transection through the medulla

chapter 2 PHYSIOLOGY

ANSWERS

1 Hypoventilation may result in:

- a **True** This may be seen in the postoperative period when the patient is experiencing the cumulative effects of the anaesthetic and analgesic drugs. Hypoventilation will produce hypoxia in the absence of supplemental oxygen.
- b **True** Respiratory acidosis is accompanied by a rise in bicarbonate levels.
- c **True** The increase in $PaCO_2$ will lead to respiratory acidosis and decreased pH.
- d **True** Alveolar ventilation may not be met during hypoventilation and may result in increased physiological dead space.
- e **True** Some patients rely on a hypoxic drive for ventilation, and giving supplemental oxygen abolishes this drive and exacerbates the hypoventilation, leading to hypercarbia.

Aitkenhead A and Smith G (2008) *Textbook of Anaesthesia*, 5th edition. Edinburgh: Churchill Livingstone.
Barrett K, Barman S, Boitano S, and Brooks HL (2009) *Ganong's Review of Medical Physiology*, 23rd edition. USA: McGraw-Hill.

2 The cough reflex:

- a **False** The vagus nerves are the afferents from the respiratory passages.
- b **False** The impulses are carried to the medulla where an automatic sequence of events occurs as follows; rapid intake of about 2.5 litres of air, closure of the glottis, forceful contraction of abdominal muscles pushing against the diaphragm, while other expiratory muscles such as the internal intercostals also contract forcefully.
- c **False** A rapid intake of approximately 2.5 litres occurs before the cough.
- d **True** Because of the closure of the glottis the pressure in the lungs increases greatly.
- e **True** The sudden and wide opening of the vocal cords makes the air under high pressure in the lungs explode outwards, thus reaching a high velocity.

Guyton A and Hall J (2000) *Textbook of Medical Physiology*, 10th edition. Philadelphia: WB Saunders.

3 Peripheral vascular resistance:

a **False** Peripheral vascular resistance is controlled mainly by the arterioles in the muscles.

b **True** The higher the peripheral resistance the greater the afterload.

c **True** Low-dose adrenaline (epinephrine) infusions have a predominant beta effect, causing fall in diastolic blood pressure and decrease in peripheral vascular resistance.

d **False** Dopamine has the effect of improving the splanchnic and renal circulations. At less than 10 μg/kg/min, it lowers peripheral vascular resistance. Higher doses cause increase in systemic vascular resistance and venous return.

e **True** Blood pressure (mean arterial pressure or MAP) is a product of the cardiac output (CO) and systemic vascular resistance (SVR): MAP = CO × SVR.

Aitkenhead A and Smith G (2008) *Textbook of Anaesthesia*, 5th edition. Edinburgh: Churchill Livingstone.

Barrett K, Barman S, Boitano S, and Brooks HL (2009) *Ganong's Review of Medical Physiology*, 23rd edition. USA: McGraw-Hill.

4 The following are produced during the synthesis or metabolism of catecholamines:

a **True** Tyrosine is first converted to DOPA, and then to dopamine, leading further to the production of noradrenaline (norepinephrine) and adrenaline (epinephrine).

b **False** 5-hydroxy indole acetic acid is a metabolite of serotonin secreted in urine.

c **False** Beta imidazole ethylamine is histamine.

d **False** Pipecolyl xylidine is a metabolic product of bupivacaine.

e **True** 3-methoxy 4-hydroxy mandelic acid is a breakdown product of noradrenaline. One test for phaeochromocytoma is the urinary estimation of this product.

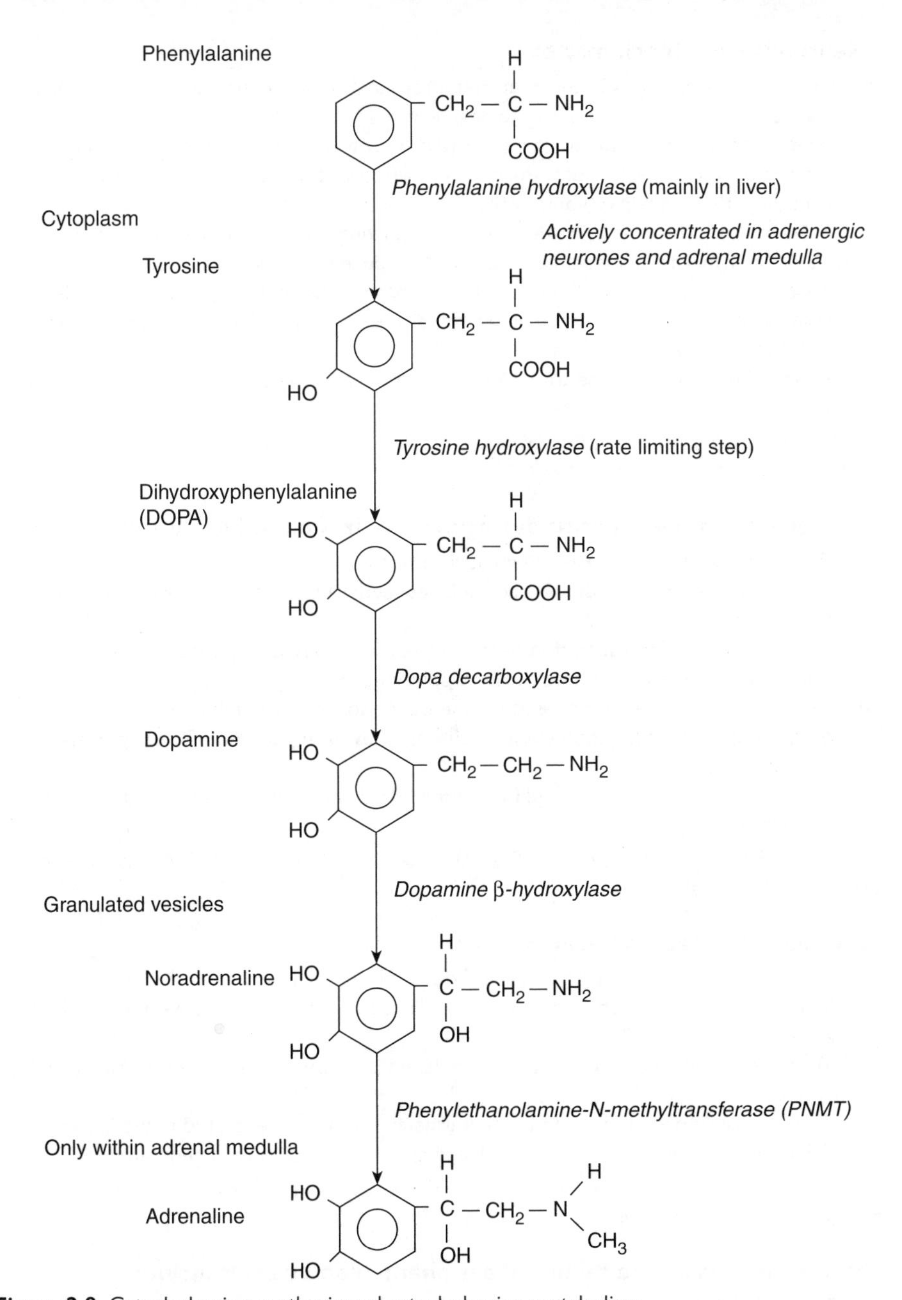

Figure 2.8 Catecholamine synthesis and catecholamine metabolism.
Reproduced with kind permission from Yentis SM, Hirsch NP and Smith GB (2004). *Anaesthesia and Intensive Care*. Edinburgh: Elsevier.

Peck T, Hill S, and Williams M (2004) *Pharmacology for Anaesthesia and Intensive Care*, 2nd edition. Cambridge: Cambridge University Press.

5 Neuromuscular block may exist:

a **True** Magnesium acts at the neuromuscular junction decreasing acetylcholine release and reducing endplate sensitivity to acetylcholine.

b **True** The botulinum exotoxin binds irreversibly to the nerve ending preventing acetylcholine release. It affects the neuromuscular junction, autonomic ganglia, and parasympathetic postganglionic fibres.

c **False** Although dysfunction due to muscle wasting and weakness is a prominent feature of hyperphosphataemia, it does not produce neuromuscular blockade.

d **True** If edrophonium does not elicit a response, it resembles a picture of muscle paralysis caused in this instance by overmedication with anticholinesterases and can be classified as a cholinergic crisis.

e **False** If there is response to both types of stimulation a neuromuscular block cannot exist.

Barrett K, Barman S, Boitano S, and Brooks HL (2009) *Ganong's Review of Medical Physiology*, 23rd edition. USA: McGraw-Hill.

6 Compensatory mechanisms during acclimatization to high altitude include:

a **False** Respiratory alkalosis is the initial response.

b **False** After a few days, the alkalaemia is reduced via increased loss of bicarbonate from the kidneys.

c **True** Erythropoietin secretion by the kidneys increases in response the low blood PO_{2}. A prolonged period at altitude causes a polycythaemia.

d **True** 2,3-DPG levels increase as compensation for hypoxia, shifting the oxyhaemoglobin dissociation curve to the right, favouring oxygen offloading to the tissues.

e **True** The adjustment in CSF pH is accomplished within 24 hours to compensate for the alkalaemia.

Pocock G and Richards C (2004) *Human Physiology: The Basis of Medicine*, 3rd edition. Oxford: Oxford University Press.

7 Breakdown of haemoglobin involves:

a **True** This is the first part of the breakdown of haemoglobin.

b **True** When haem is broken down biliverdin is formed, which is converted to bilirubin and excreted in the bile.

c **True** Another significant component of haem is iron, which is reused for haemoglobin synthesis.

d **True** Urobilinogen is excreted in the urine and urobilin is excreted in the faeces.

e **False** When carbon monoxide is inhaled carboxyhaemoglobin is generated.

Barrett K, Barman S, Boitano S, and Brooks HL (2009) *Ganong's Review of Medical Physiology*, 23rd edition. USA: McGraw-Hill.

8 Factors increasing the calibre of peripheral blood vessels include:

a **False** Hypothermia produces vasoconstriction.

b **True** Hypoxia increases the calibre of arterioles in the periphery. In the pulmonary circulation hypoxia produces vasoconstriction.

c **False** Alkalosis produces vasoconstriction.

d **False** Serotonin causes vasoconstriction.

e **True** Respiratory acidosis causes arteriolar dilation.

Barrett K, Barman S, Boitano S, and Brooks HL (2009) *Ganong's Review of Medical Physiology*, 23rd edition. USA: McGraw-Hill.

9 Concerning carbohydrate metabolism:

a **False** Fructose is phosphorylated to fructose 6-phosphate then to fructose 1,6-diphosphate in the absence of insulin, and it enters the Embden–Meyerhof pathway independently. Dihydroxyacetone phosphate and glyceraldehyde are other products of phosphorylation that can similarly enter the metabolic pathway.

b **False** During aerobic glycolysis 38 moles of ATP are produced.

c **True** Gluconeogenesis is the term for generation of glucose from non-carbohydrate sources, e.g. amino acids, lactate, and glycerol.

d **False** Glycogenolysis is the conversion of glycogen to glucose in the liver and skeletal muscle.

e **True** 50% of ingested glucose is burned to CO_2 and H_2O, 5% is converted to glycogen and 30–40% is converted to fat.

Barrett K, Barman S, Boitano S, and Brooks HL (2009) *Ganong's Review of Medical Physiology*, 23rd edition. USA: McGraw-Hill.

10 The tracts in the spinal cord serve the following functions:

a **False** Lateral spinothalamic tract is the main carrier of pain and temperature. It occupies the lateral white substance of the spinal cord and continues to the thalamus on the opposite side.

b **True** The posterior columns carry ipsilateral touch, vibration, and proprioception from the lower body via the fasciculus gracilis and from the upper body via the fasciculus cuneatus, uncrossed to the medulla.

c **False** The anterior spinothalamic tract carries contralateral touch and pressure sensations only. The lateral spinothalamic tract conveys contralateral pain and temperature sensation.

d **False** The fasciculus gracilis in the posterior column carries ipsilateral touch, vibration, and proprioception from the lower body.

e **True** The crossed motor tract commences in the pyramidal cells of the motor cortex, decussates in the medulla, and descends in the pyramidal tract on the contralateral side of the cord.

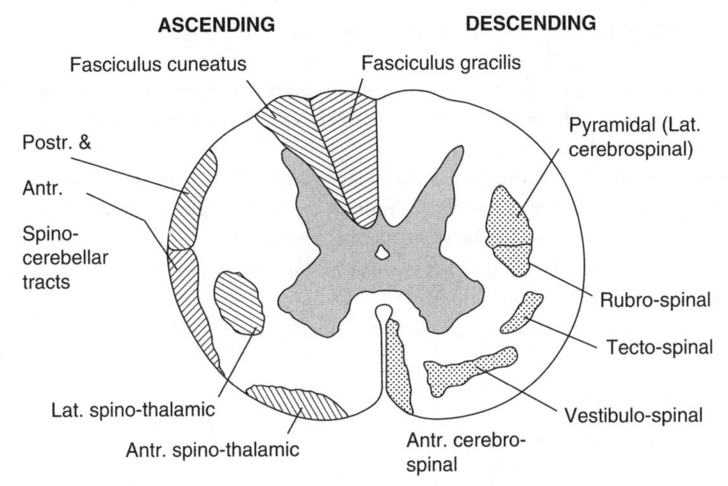

Figure 2.9 Transverse section of the thoracic cord showing the spinal tracts.
Reproduced with kind permission from Ellis H, Feldman S and Griffiths W (2004) *Anatomy for anaesthetists*, 8th edition. Oxford: Wiley Blackwell.

Ellis H, Feldman S, and Griffiths W (2004) *Anatomy for anaesthetists*, 8th edition. Oxford: Wiley Blackwell.

11 The following are cholinergic:

a **True** Preganglionic sympathetic fibres are cholinergic.
b **True** The preganglionic fibres to the adrenal medulla are cholinergic.
c **True** Although the fibres originate in the sympathetic system, they release acetylcholine in their nerve endings.
d **False** Postganglionic sympathetic fibres release noradrenaline (norepinephrine).
e **True** The supply is from the second to fourth sacral segments.

Barrett K, Barman S, Boitano S, and Brooks HL (2009) *Ganong's Review of Medical Physiology*, 23rd edition. USA: McGraw-Hill.

12 The transmission of nerve impulses is:

a **True** Conduction in myelinated fibres jumps from one node of Ranvier to the next and is described as saltatory conduction, which is 50 times faster than conduction in any non-myelinated nerve.
b **True** Reduction in potassium bathing the outside of the nerve membrane reduces the rate of pumping of sodium ions.
c **True** A current strong enough and of sufficient duration will elicit a response.
d **True** For nerve transmission to occur, production of ATP is necessary to activate the sodium pump. Hence during maximal activity the metabolism in the nerve may double.
e **True** The synapses do not allow retrograde conduction.

Barrett K, Barman S, Boitano S, and Brooks HL (2009) *Ganong's Review of Medical Physiology*, 23rd edition. USA: McGraw-Hill.

13 Cerebral blood flow:

a **False** Mean cerebral blood flow to the adult brain is around 50 ml/100 g/min or approximately 700 ml/min.
b **False** It is not increased during mental activity and remains the same or even increased during sleep.
c **True** The grey matter receives more than twice (70 ml/100 g/min) the blood flow than the white matter (30 ml/100 g/min).
d **True** Although the cerebral vessels are innervated by adrenergic vasoconstrictor and parasympathetic dilator fibres, vasomotor reflexes play little part in the regulation of cerebral blood flow in humans.
e **False** Positive 'G' with sudden ascent leads to blood flow towards the feet, eventually causing loss of vision as a 'black out'. Sudden descent produces negative 'G', which causes blood to be directed to the head, producing a 'red out'.

Pinnock C, Lin T, and Smith T (2002) *Fundamentals of Anaesthesia*, 2nd edition. New York: Cambridge University Press.
Pocock G and Richards C (2004) *Human Physiology: The basis of medicine*, 3rd edition. Oxford: Oxford University Press.

14 Haemoglobin:

a **True** Each subunit has a molecular weight of 16 000–17 000 daltons, giving a molecular weight of 64 000–68 000 daltons.
b **True** It has about 210 times more affinity for carbon monoxide than oxygen.
c **False** Fetal haemoglobin has two alpha and two gamma chains.
d **False** It is a combination of HbS and HbA. HbSS in sickle cell disease and HbAS in sickle cell trait.
e **True** The dissolved oxygen is directly dependent on the partial pressure of oxygen. Under hyperbaric oxygen therapy the dissolved oxygen content would be increased to such an extent that the tissue needs can be met entirely by dissolved oxygen. Therefore the haemoglobin does not release its oxygen. This has been cited as one of the causes of convulsions during hyperbaric oxygen therapy. Fully oxygenated haemoglobin is incapable of acting as an efficient buffer and consequently there is a build up of metabolic products of tissue respiration. This interferes with normal neuronal function producing convulsions.

Barrett K, Barman S, Boitano S, and Brooks HL (2009) *Ganong's Review of Medical Physiology*, 23rd edition. USA: McGraw-Hill.
Pocock G and Richards C (2004) *Human Physiology: The Basis of Medicine*, 3rd edition. Oxford: Oxford University Press.

15 Concerning renal function:

a **True** Although such a large volume is filtered, only 1–1.5 litres of urine are excreted in 24 hours.
b **False** Active reabsorption of sodium occurs in the proximal tubule. This sets up an osmotic gradient, which causes passive water reabsorption.
c **True** Specific gravity of urine may vary with the constituents within it. For example a patient excreting a radio-labelled marker after a scan may have urine specific gravity of 1.04–1.05 with very little rise in osmolality. Hence it is more accurate to measure osmolality.
d **True** Although 100 mg/min of glucose is filtered through the glomerulus, almost all of it is reabsorbed, leaving only a few milligrams in the urine per 24 hours.
e **False** If the substance is also secreted by the renal tubules, the clearance would exceed the glomerular filtration rate.

Barrett K, Barman S, Boitano S, and Brooks HL (2009) *Ganong's Review of Medical Physiology*, 23rd edition. USA: McGraw-Hill.

16 Concerning the adrenal gland:

a **True** Preganglionic fibres to the sympathetic system are cholinergic.
b **True** In an unstressed individual, production of cortisol is approximately 20 mg/day.
c **False** Normal aldosterone secretion is 0.15 mg/day.
d **False** Metyrapone inhibits 11-beta hydroxylase, and the resultant cortisol deficiency stimulates the pituitary to increase adrenocorticotropic hormone (ACTH) secretion. It is used as a test of pituitary reserve.
e **False** Androgens secreted by the adrenal gland are only 20% as effective as testosterone produced by the testes, and the quantity produced is insignificant compared to testicular production.

Barrett K, Barman S, Boitano S, and Brooks HL (2009) *Ganong's Review of Medical Physiology*, 23rd edition. USA: McGraw-Hill.

17 In nerve muscle physiology:

a **False** Chronaxie is the shortest time interval during which a current twice the strength of a rheobase should be passed to elicit a response.

b **False** Gamma efferent motor fibres to muscle spindles act to pre-tension the muscle, setting its sensitivity. High gamma efferent tone means muscle spindles are taut and slight variation in muscle length elicits a contraction. The opposite is seen with low gamma efferent tone.

c **True** Normal resting membrane potential is –70 mV, being more negative inside the nerve.

d **True** During an action potential, there is an increase in sodium conduction, sodium ions diffuse down their electrochemical gradients so that the inside of the neurone becomes more positive, to a peak of +35 mV.

e **False** During the absolute refractory period no response is elicited. During the relative refractory period, a supra-maximal stimulus is necessary produce excitation.

Barrett K, Barman S, Boitano S, and Brooks HL (2009) *Ganong's Review of Medical Physiology*, 23rd edition. USA: McGraw-Hill.

18 Hypercarbia:

a **False** Bicarbonate levels increase in respiratory acidosis by means of compensation.

b **True** A normal PO_2 can exist in the presence of hypercarbia if oxygen is administered to a patient who is hypoventilating. This is the reason that oxygen saturations can give false reassurance as to a patient's condition. Once the hypoxic drive is completely removed apnoea would occur.

c **True** The initial rise in catecholamines in response to hypercarbia produces a bounding pulse, increased blood pressure, and a pink colour. After a while catecholamines produce a mottled and sweaty appearance and cardiac arrhythmias occur as a result of sensitization of the myocardium.

d **True** The cerebral circulation is increased as a result of vasodilation. For this reason it is important to control the $PaCO_2$ in a head injured patient in order to prevent secondary brain injury.

e **False** The pH decreases with respiratory acidosis.

Barrett K, Barman S, Boitano S, and Brooks HL (2009) *Ganong's Review of Medical Physiology*, 23rd edition. USA: McGraw-Hill.

19 Concerning renal physiology:

a **True** The GFR falls less than the RPF during hypotension, and the filtration fraction consequently rises, which is observed early in congestive cardiac failure and may account for the salt and water retention.

b **True** The total filtration in 24 hours is 180 litres at this rate but only just over a litre of urine is passed daily. Thus over 99% of all the filtrate is reabsorbed.

c **True** Approximately 12 mmol of creatinine is filtered over 24 hours and none is reabsorbed.

d **True** The pressure in the glomerular capillary is 50 mmHg, which has to overcome the hydrostatic pressure of 10 mmHg and plasma oncotic pressure of 25 mmHg, giving an effective filtration pressure of 15 mmHg.

e **True** Carbonic anhydrase is essential for converting carbonic acid to hydrogen ions and bicarbonate.

Barrett K, Barman S, Boitano S, and Brooks HL (2009) *Ganong's Review of Medical Physiology*, 23rd edition. USA: McGraw-Hill.

20 The following are normal values in the cardiovascular system:

a **True** A left atrial pressure of 4–12 mmHg is normal.
b **False** Right ventricular pressure could rise up to 30 mmHg.
c **False** End-systolic ventricular volume is 50 ml. At end diastole the volume is in the region of 120 ml or more during normal activity.
d **True** A time interval of 0.12–0.2 seconds is considered normal.
e **True** Ventricular systole lasts for 0.3 seconds and diastole for 0.5 seconds.

Barrett K, Barman S, Boitano S, and Brooks HL (2009) *Ganong's Review of Medical Physiology*, 23rd edition. USA: McGraw-Hill.

21 Coronary blood flow:

a **True** Since the blood flow occurs mainly during diastole, the mean pressure is a better guide to coronary perfusion than systolic pressure.
b **False** During isovolumetric contraction the blood vessels in the myocardium are compressed, and therefore the flow is greater at the end of systole into diastole.
c **True** Sympathetic stimulation improves the cardiac output and thus increases the coronary flow as well. However, at very high heart rates diastolic time is decreased and coronary blood flow is reduced.
d **True** Acute hypoxia causes vasodilation of the coronary blood vessels and therefore can increase coronary blood flow by 200–300%.
e **True** At rest normal coronary blood flow is 250 ml/min or 84 ml/100 g/min.

Barrett K, Barman S, Boitano S, and Brooks HL (2009) *Ganong's Review of Medical Physiology*, 23rd edition. USA: McGraw-Hill.
Pocock G and Richards C (2004) *Human Physiology: The Basis of Medicine*, 3rd edition. Oxford: Oxford University Press.

22 2,3-DPG:

a **True** The dissociation curve is shifted to the right when 2,3-DPG levels increase.
b **True** Thyroid hormone, growth hormone, and androgens are known to increase 2,3-DPG levels.
c **False** 2,3-DPG levels are increased in anaemia to counteract the chronic hypoxia.
d **True** The levels rise within 60 minutes of exercise.
e **True** 2,3-DPG is not well preserved in stored blood. However levels are better preserved in SAGM blood (saline, adenine, glucose, mannitol) compared to blood preserved with CPD (citrate phosphate dextrose) and ACD (acid citrate dextrose).

Barrett K, Barman S, Boitano S, and Brooks HL (2009) *Ganong's Review of Medical Physiology*, 23rd edition. USA: McGraw-Hill.

23 In a patient with obstructive airway disease:

a **False** The lung compliance may be normal or raised.
b **True** Since it may be difficult to perform the test adequately, all the volumes tested would be low.
c **True** FEV_1 is reduced, and the ratio of FEV_1/FVC is <80%.
d **True** As maximal voluntary ventilation is derived from $35 \times FEV_1$ this will also be reduced.
e **True** In obstructive airway disease, expiration is limited and PEFR is reduced.

Barrett K, Barman S, Boitano S, and Brooks HL (2009) *Ganong's Review of Medical Physiology*, 23rd edition. USA: McGraw-Hill.

24 Plasma proteins:

a **True** Plasma proteins are albumin (35–50 g/l) and globulins (25–35 g/l).
b **True** The most important protein is albumin, which contributes 75% of the total osmotic pressure.
c **False** Plasma proteins are the main intracellular buffers. For example in metabolic acidosis 15–20% is buffered in the blood by haemoglobin, 20–25% is buffered by the carbonic acid-bicarbonate system in the interstitial fluid, and the rest is buffered by plasma proteins.
d **False** Albumin is filtered (mw 65 000 daltons) in small quantities but is normally reabsorbed in the proximal tubules.
e **True** Thyroxine is bound to albumin and adrenocorticoids are bound to alpha globulin.

Barrett K, Barman S, Boitano S, and Brooks HL (2009) *Ganong's Review of Medical Physiology*, 23rd edition. USA: McGraw-Hill.

25 In the coagulation system:

a **False** Tissue thromboplastins are an important source in the extrinsic pathway of coagulation.
b **True** Platelets detect damaged endothelium and adhere to it. They release their contents including serotonin and ADP, which aid platelet aggregation. When enough platelets have collected together they form a plug, preventing further blood loss through the vessel wall.
c **False** Plasmin, also known as fibrinolysin, acts on the formed clot fibrin to disrupt the clotting mechanism.
d **False** Factor XI features in the intrinsic pathway only.
e **False** Factor X, also known as the Stuart–Prower factor, is not responsible for haemophilia. It is the deficiency of factor VIII or IX which is responsible for haemophilia A and B, respectively.

Barrett K, Barman S, Boitano S, and Brooks HL (2009) *Ganong's Review of Medical Physiology*, 23rd edition. USA: McGraw-Hill.
Pocock G and Richards C (2004) *Human Physiology: The basis of medicine*, 3rd edition. Oxford: Oxford University Press.

26 Regarding temperature regulation:

a **True** In addition, neurones within the septal area of the hypothalamus and the reticular substance of the midbrain also have a role.
b **True** In addition there are peripheral thermoreceptors in the skin and elsewhere which relay information to the thermoregulatory centre.
c **True** The rectal temperature is also higher than the oral temperature due to bacterial fermentation.
d **True** A diurnal variation in temperature (0.5–0.7 °C) exists in the normal individuals, being lowest at night and highest in mid afternoon.
e **True** TSH secretion is increased by exposure to cold and depressed by heat.

Barrett K, Barman S, Boitano S, and Brooks HL (2009) *Ganong's Review of Medical Physiology*, 23rd edition. USA: McGraw-Hill.

27 The pupillary light reflex:

a **False** The oculomotor nerve is the efferent pathway for the light reflex.

b **True** When both pupils constrict in response to light on one eye, it confirms the integrity of the oculomotor nerves.

c **True** In the Argyll Robertson pupil, which is a feature of neurosyphilis, the light reflex is absent but the accommodation reflex is present. (The initials AR (Argyll Robertson) serves as a reminder that accommodation reflex is present, and light reflex is not).

d **True** The impulse travels through the optic nerve, optic chiasma, and optic tract to the lateral geniculate bodies until it synapses at the Edinger–Westphal nucleus of the third cranial nerve situated at superior colliculus in the midbrain. The fibres also cross to the nucleus on the other side, producing the consensual reflex. From the mid-brain the impulse travels through the oculomotor nerve to the ciliary ganglion and thence through short ciliary nerves to the pupil.

e **False** Short ciliary nerves carry the impulse to the iris sphincter muscles on both sides causing pupil constriction.

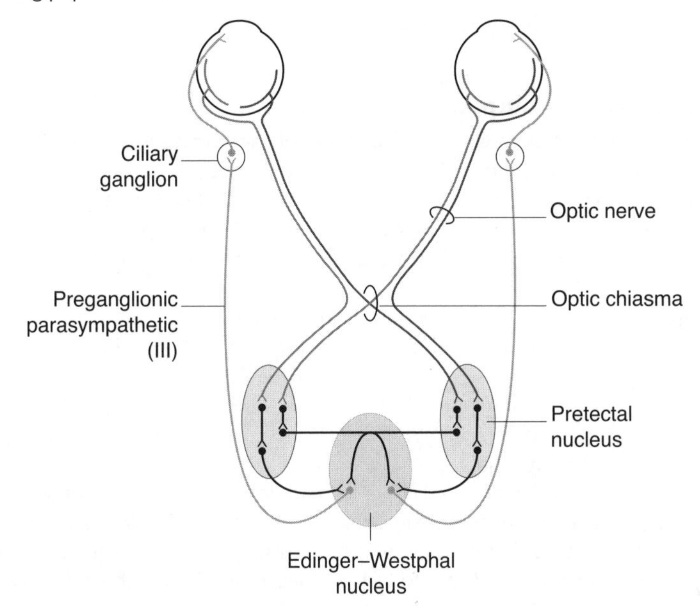

Figure 2.10 The light reflex.
Reproduced with kind permission from Kevin K and Spoors C (2009) *Training in Anaesthesia*. New York: Oxford University Press.

Barrett K, Barman S, Boitano S, and Brooks HL (2009) *Ganong's Review of Medical Physiology*, 23rd edition. USA: McGraw-Hill.
Kevin K and Spoors C (2009) *Training in Anaesthesia*. New York: Oxford University Press.
Pocock G and Richards C (2004) *Human Physiology: The basis of medicine*, 3rd edition. Oxford: Oxford University Press.

28 Among the cranial nerves:

a **True** Because of its long intracranial course, the abducens nerve is frequently involved in injuries to the base of skull. When damaged or stretched, it causes diplopia and a convergent squint.

b **True** It supplies all eye muscles except lateral rectus and superior oblique. In addition, it conveys the parasympathetic preganglionic fibres for the sphincter of the pupil and for the ciliary muscle.

c **True** The oculo-cardiac reflex is mediated through the ophthalmic division of the trigeminal nerve (afferent) and the vagus (efferent), producing bradycardia in response to traction on extraocular muscles, e.g. during squint surgery or blunt injury that has even resulted in death among boxers.

d **True** The glossopharyngeal nerve also supplies the posterior third of the tongue. The posterior surface of the epiglottis is supplied by the internal laryngeal branch of the superior laryngeal nerve, a branch of the vagus.

e **True** It is the only cranial nerve in the neck that is purely motor.

Ellis H, Feldman S, and Griffiths W (2004) *Anatomy for Anaesthetists*, 8th edition. Oxford: Wiley Blackwell.

29 Concerning cardiac output:

a **True** The heart rate can be increased threefold and stroke volume is able to double to meet the increased demands during strenuous exercise.

b **False** The stroke volume at rest is approximately 70–80 ml in an adult.

c **True** In trained athletes the resting stroke volume is high, up to 120 ml, hence they have the reserve to raise their cardiac output to >35 l/min during heavy exercise.

d **True**

$$\text{CO (l/min)} = \frac{\text{oxygen uptake (ml/min)}}{\text{arterial–mixed venous } O_2 \text{ concentration (ml/l)}}$$

for example:

$$\frac{250 \text{ ml/min}}{200 - 150 \text{ ml/l}}$$

$$= 5 \text{ l/min.}$$

e **False** On exercise there is initially an increase in venous return causing stretching of the cardiac fibres and an increase in stroke volume via the Frank–Starling relationship. The cardiac output is therefore increased. Circulating catecholamines are also able to have a direct effect on the heart to increase heart rate despite the lack of sympathetic innervations. These changes occur in sequence in contrast to the non-transplanted heart, where these changes occur simultaneously.

Barrett K, Barman S, Boitano S, and Brooks HL (2009) *Ganong's Review of Medical Physiology*, 23rd edition. USA: McGraw-Hill.

30 In control of respiration:

a **True** The apneustic centre in the lower pons causes excitation of medullary inspiratory neurones. Transection above it causes prolonged inspiratory gasping. If the vagus is also divided this produces apneusis (breath held at end inspiration).

b **True** The response to hypoxia only occurs at lower levels, i.e. less than 7–8 kPa.

c **True** The inspiratory muscles are inhibited after lung inflation. The reflex is possibly mediated by pulmonary stretch receptors via the vagus. This reflex is more important in other mammals.

d **True** In any situation which may cause hypoxia the carotid and aortic bodies stimulate an increase in respiration.

e **False** Kussmaul respiration or air hunger describes the rapid deep respiration originally associated with diabetic ketoacidosis. It can be associated with severe metabolic acidosis of any cause where the low pH stimulates the respiratory centre.

Barrett K, Barman S, Boitano S, and Brooks HL (2009) *Ganong's Review of Medical Physiology*, 23rd edition. USA: McGraw-Hill.

chapter 3

PHARMACOLOGY

QUESTIONS

1 Fentanyl:

a Is a synthetic phenyl piperidine derivative
b Has a duration of action of 10–15 minutes
c Is mainly excreted unchanged by the kidney
d May produce an increase in expiratory muscle tone
e May cause late-onset respiratory depression

2 The following should be avoided in patients susceptible to malignant hyperpyrexia:

a Suxamethonium
b Thiopental (thiopentone)
c Propofol
d Atracurium
e Fentanyl

3 Monoamine oxidase inhibitors (MAOIs):

a May cause a type I reaction known as 'serotonin syndrome'
b Inhibit hepatic microsomal enzymes and potentiate all opioid effects (type II reaction)
c All cause a decrease in plasma pseudocholinesterase
d Cause severe hypertension with the use of pancuronium
e Should be discontinued for one week prior to anaesthesia

4 Drugs producing antiarrhythmic action by altering sodium permeability include:

a Lidocaine (lignocaine)
b Propranolol
c Quinidine
d Phenytoin
e Digoxin

5 Tricyclic antidepressants:

a Are also known as selective serotonin reuptake inhibitors (SSRIs)
b Action may be enhanced by being displaced from protein-binding sites by aspirin
c Are used in the treatment of chronic pain
d May cause hyponatraemia
e Have a clinical effect after 48 hours of administration

6 Lithium:

a Increases the release of central neurotransmitters
b Toxicity occurs at plasma levels of >2.5 mmol/l
c Potentiates neuromuscular blocking drugs
d Overdose produces a prominent T wave on the electrocardiogram (ECG)
e May trigger neuroleptic malignant syndrome

7 Drugs to be used with caution in epilepsy include:

a Methohexitone
b Ketamine
c Tramadol
d Ondansetron
e Propofol

8 Drugs considered safe in chronic renal failure include:

a Pethidine
b Enflurane
c Pancuronium
d Sevoflurane
e Midazolam

9 Concerning warfarin:

a It is structurally related to bishydroxyl coumarin
b It interferes with factors II, VII, IX, and X to produce its effects
c It is teratogenic
d The peak concentration in blood occurs an hour after ingestion, and coincides with the peak pharmacological effect
e Its action is potentiated by phenytoin

10 One litre of Gelofusine® contains:

a Na^+ 131 mmol
b Cl^- 112 mmol
c K^+ 3 mmol
d Ca^{2+} 5 mmol
e Mg^{2+} 2 mmol

11 Angiotensin-converting enzyme (ACE) inhibitors:

a Inhibit conversion of angiotensin I to angiotensin II
b Are usually used along with diuretics
c Lower the blood pressure gradually
d When administered with non-steroidal anti-inflammatory drugs (NSAIDs) can produce renal damage
e May cause angioedema

12 Regarding local anaesthetic toxicity:

- a Brachial plexus block is more likely to predispose to toxicity than a caudal block
- b Respiratory acidosis increases the risk of toxicity
- c Symptoms of impending toxicity are different for esters and amides
- d Cardiovascular effects usually occur before neurological effects
- e Lipid emulsion forms part of the management of cardiac arrest secondary to local anaesthetic toxicity

13 Bicarbonate (HCO_3^-):

- a Infusion is used to treat metabolic acidosis
- b Is hypotonic in relation to blood
- c 8.4% solution contains 8.4 mg/ml
- d Administration shifts the oxyhaemoglobin dissociation curve to the left
- e Added to local anaesthetic drugs enhances their duration of action

14 One litre of Hartmann's solution contains:

- a Na^+ 154 mmol
- b Cl^- 154 mmol
- c Lactate 29 mmol
- d K^+ 2.5 mmol
- e Ca^{2+} 5.0 mmol

15 Hyoscine:

- a Is a natural alkaloid of the plant family Solanaceae (night shade)
- b Is antiemetic
- c Causes less mental confusion than atropine
- d Can increase pyrexia
- e Is used to reduce intestinal motility

16 Antifibrinolytic agents include:

- a Epsilon-amino caproic acid
- b Mefenamic acid
- c Tranexamic acid
- d Streptokinase
- e Desmopressin

17 Angiotensin II receptor antagonists:

- a Have many properties similar to ACE inhibitors
- b Inhibit the breakdown of bradykinin
- c Potentiate muscle relaxants
- d Typically cause hypokalaemia
- e May have a 24-hour half-life

18 Regarding local anaesthetic drugs:

- a The first local anaesthetic drug to be used clinically was procaine
- b Dibucaine is the drug used in the pseudocholinesterase assay
- c Prilocaine is currently used for topical anaesthesia
- d Bupivacaine has a lower pKa than lidocaine (lignocaine)
- e Amethocaine lozenges are used to anaesthetize the oropharynx prior to upper gastrointestinal endoscopy

19 NSAIDs:

- a Are cyclo-oxygenase (COX) inhibitors
- b Impair platelet function
- c Have an opioid-sparing effect of between 50% and 60%
- d With sole COX-2 inhibition have no action on the gastric mucosa
- e Should be avoided in renal impairment

20 Sugammadex:

- a Is a modified gamma-cyclodextrin
- b Can be used to antagonize suxamethonium
- c Cannot reverse an intubating dose of rocuronium until two twitches are seen on train-of-four monitoring
- d Is only able to reverse the action of rocuronium
- e Is contraindicated in diabetic patients

21 Metoclopramide:

- a Is a dopamine receptor antagonist
- b Increases gastric motility and emptying
- c Relaxes the lower oesophageal sphincter
- d May stimulate lactation
- e Is associated with extrapyramidal side effects

22 Concerning cholinesterase and anticholinesterases:

- a Acetylcholinesterase is bound to the basement membrane in the synaptic cleft
- b Plasma cholinesterase is also known as butyryl cholinesterase
- c Neostigmine is a medium-acting anticholinesterase
- d Ecothiopate is used as eye drops
- e Organophosphorous poisoning enhances the action of acetylcholinesterase

23 Low molecular weight heparins (LMWHs):

- a Increase the action of antithrombin III (AT III) on factor Xa
- b Are more effective than unfractionated heparin in forming the 'antithrombin III–thrombin' complex
- c Have a longer half-life than fractionated heparin
- d Are mainly eliminated by the liver
- e Prolong the activated partial thromboplastin time (APTT)

24 Protamine:

a Is extracted from sperm cells of salmon
b Is chemically basic in nature
c Is associated with allergic reactions
d May provoke severe hypertension
e Can cause bleeding if given in excessive doses

25 Cisatracurium:

a Is an isomer of atracurium
b Has a duration of action of over 60 minutes
c Action is potentiated by metabolic alkalosis
d Has an initial intubating (loading) dose, similar to atracurium, of 0.5 mg/kg
e Causes less histamine release than atracurium

26 Vecuronium:

a Is an aminosteroid
b Has an average duration of action of 55 minutes
c Causes bradycardia
d Is dependent on renal excretion
e Has an active metabolite

27 Metaraminol:

a Is a pure alpha adrenergic agonist
b Causes tachycardia
c Has a duration of action of 60–75 minutes when given IV
d Decreases the placental circulation
e Should be avoided in hyperthyroidism

28 Phentolamine:

a Is an alpha 1 and alpha 2 antagonist
b May be used in phaeochromocytoma management
c Causes bradycardia
d May cause nasal stuffiness
e Related hypotension should be treated with adrenaline (epinephrine)

29 Amethocaine:

a Is also known as tetracaine
b Is the main component of the topical gel Ametop®
c Was the first amide local anaesthetic to be used
d Is associated with methaemoglobinaemia
e Is also available as eye drops

30 Drugs to be avoided in asthma include:

a Etomidate
b Suxamethonium
c Ketamine
d Rocuronium
e Pethidine

chapter 3 PHARMACOLOGY

ANSWERS

1 Fentanyl:

- a **True** It is a derivative of pethidine.
- b **False** Its peak effect is at four to five minutes, and its duration of action is 20 minutes until it is redistributed.
- c **False** It is extensively metabolized in the liver. Only 10% is excreted unchanged.
- d **True** As with other piperidine derivatives, increase in expiratory muscle tone is observed frequently when high doses are used or an intravenous infusion of the drug is being used.
- e **True** When fentanyl has been used either by the subarachnoid or the epidural route, caution should be observed with administration of other opiates in the postoperative period. Respiratory depression can also result from a cumulative effect of the drug if a relatively large initial dose was used.

Aitkenhead A and Smith G (2008) *Textbook of Anaesthesia*, 5th edition. Edinburgh: Churchill Livingstone.
Allman K and Wilson I (2006) *Oxford Handbook of Anaesthesia*, 2nd edition. New York: Oxford University Press.

2 The following should be avoided in malignant hyperpyrexia susceptible patients:

- a **True** Suxamethonium is a prominent trigger agent for malignant hyperpyrexia, along with the inhalational agents, particularly halothane. Insufficient relaxation with suxamethonium and the presence of masseter spasm may be associated with susceptibility to malignant hyperpyrexia.
- b **False** There is no known association between any of the IV induction agents and malignant hyperpyrexia.
- c **False** Propofol and other agents can be used as total intravenous anaesthesia (TIVA) for cases with suspected or confirmed malignant hyperpyrexia.
- d **False** Atracurium is safe, as are all of the non-depolarizing neuromuscular blocking drugs.
- e **False** All analgesic drugs are safe in malignant hyperpyrexia.

Allman K and Wilson I (2006) *Oxford Handbook of Anaesthesia*, 2nd edition. New York: Oxford University Press.

3 Monoamine oxidase inhibitors (MAOIs):

a **True** It is caused by increased synaptic levels of serotonin in the brain stem and the spinal cord and presents with central nervous system (CNS) excitation, muscular rigidity, and autonomic instability.

b **True** This potentiation can be reversed with naloxone.

c **False** Only one of the MAOI drugs, phenelzine, has this effect of lowering pseudocholinesterase levels. It is not typical of the other MAOI drugs.

d **True** Pancuronium depletes the adrenaline (epinephrine) and noradrenaline (norepinephrine) stores from nerve endings and is responsible for hypertension with normal use. In combination with MAOI drugs this would be even more dramatic.

e **False** Traditionally, MAOIs were discontinued three weeks prior to elective surgery. However, this is no longer advised as there is a risk of severe depression recurring and the washout period may be inadequate.

Allman K and Wilson I (2006) *Oxford Handbook of Anaesthesia*, 2nd edition. New York: Oxford University Press.

4 Drugs producing antiarrhythmic action by altering sodium permeability include:

a **True** Lidocaine (lignocaine) is less effective than other agents. It belongs to class 1b of the Vaughan Williams classification of antiarrhythmic drugs. Lidocaine works as an antiarrhythmic by sodium channel blockade and shortens the length of the refractory period.

b **False** Beta blockers are class II antiarrhythmics and act via direct beta adrenoceptor blockade.

c **True** Quinidine is a class Ia antiarrhythmic and works by sodium channel blockade, prolonging the cardiac muscle refractory period.

d **True** Phenytoin like lidocaine is a class 1b antiarrhythmic drug.

e **False** Digoxin has direct and indirect actions on the heart. It directly binds to and inhibits Na+/K+ ATPase, increasing intracellular sodium ions and decreasing potassium ions. These changes increase intracellular calcium ions, causing positive inotropy. Indirectly, digoxin lowers the heart rate by increasing acetylcholine release at cardiac muscarinic receptors.

Table 3.1 Vaughn–Williams classification of antiarrhythmics

Class	Action	Drug
Class I	Na channel blockers	
Ia	ADP prolonged	Procainamide
Ib	ADP shortened	Lidocaine
Ic	ADP unchanged	Flecanide
		Propafenone
Class II	β blockers	Esmolol
		Metoprolol
Class III	K channel blockers	Amiodorone
		Sotalol
Class IV	Ca channel blockers	Verapamil
		Diltiazem

ADP, adenosine diphosphate.

Peck T, Hill S, and Williams M (2004) *Pharmacology for Anaesthesia and Intensive Care*, 2nd edition. Cambridge: Cambridge University Press.

5 Tricyclic antidepressants:

a **False** SSRIs are a separate group by themselves and are less toxic than tricyclic antidepressants.
b **True** Digoxin and warfarin are other drugs that may act similarly.
c **True** They are particularly helpful in neuropathic pain, e.g. trigeminal neuralgia.
d **True** Hyponatraemia can be caused by inhibition of the sodium pump.
e **False** The drugs have to be taken for two to four weeks before they become effective.

Allman K and Wilson I (2006) *Oxford Handbook of Anaesthesia*, 2nd edition. New York: Oxford University Press.
Peck T, Hill S, and Williams M (2004) *Pharmacology for Anaesthesia and Intensive Care*, 2nd edition. Cambridge: Cambridge University Press.

6 Lithium:

a **False** Lithium reduces the release of central and peripheral neurotransmitters. It appears to mimic sodium and enters cells during depolarization, having a membrane-stabilizing effect.
b **False** Lithium toxicity occurs at levels >1.5 mmol/l. Monitoring of plasma concentrations of the drug is therefore important.
c **True** Both depolarizing and non-depolarizing relaxants are potentiated by lithium.
d **False** T wave flattening is associated with the hypokalaemia seen with standard administration. In overdose there may also be arrhythmias.
e **True** It is a rare idiosyncratic reaction, resembling malignant hyperthermia. Hyperthermia, tachycardia, and extrapyramidal dysfunction are common features.

Allman K and Wilson I (2006) *Oxford Handbook of Anaesthesia*, 2nd edition. New York: Oxford University Press.

7 Drugs to be used with caution in epilepsy include:

a **True** Methohexitone was a popular agent for short procedures, e.g. dental anaesthesia, but produces epileptiform activity in the brain. This is believed to be due to the methyl group in its structure. Some anaesthetists use methohexitone when anaesthetizing for electroconvulsive therapy (ECT) because of its ability to reduce the seizure threshold.
b **True** Owing to its CNS excitatory effects, it is suggested that ketamine is used with caution in patients with epilepsy.
c **True** Tramadol has caused convulsions, especially when administered with SSRIs or MAOIs.
d **True** Ondansetron has been known to cause convulsions and is to be used with caution in epilepsy.
e **False** Although propofol can produce jerking movements, it is also used as a sedative agent in the management of status epilepticus.

Allman K and Wilson I (2006) *Oxford Handbook of Anaesthesia*, 2nd edition. New York: Oxford University Press.

8 Drugs considered safe in chronic renal failure include:

a **False** Norpethidine, a metabolite of pethidine can accumulate and cause convulsions.

b **True** Enflurane has been avoided because of fluoride ion formation, however, during clinical use fluoride ions are not detectable in plasma in significant amounts.

c **False** It is one of the drugs that should be avoided. Although a dual pathway of elimination, i.e. hepatic and renal for pancuronium, has been suggested, in clinical practice more incidents of prolonged curarization have been reported with its use in patients with impaired renal function.

d **True** Sevoflurane is safe to use. There have been concerns regarding the formation of compound A, which causes renal failure in rats, but plasma levels in humans do not reach toxic levels.

e **True** Midazolam is safe to use with an adjustment in the dose, especially if infusions are used.

Allman K and Wilson I (2006) *Oxford Handbook of Anaesthesia*, 2nd edition. New York: Oxford University Press.

9 Concerning warfarin:

a **True** In 1920, sweet clover was substituted for corn in cattle feed in the USA, and an epidemic of haemorrhagic cattle deaths ensued. This was found to be caused by bishydroxyl coumarin in the spoiled clover and led to the discovery of warfarin. The name comes from Wisconsin Alumni Research Foundation, where warfarin was developed.

b **True** Warfarin competes with vitamin K in the synthesis of clotting factors II, VII, IX, and X in the liver.

c **True** Warfarin is avoided in early pregnancy except in some very high risk cases, e.g. patients with metallic heart valves.

d **False** Although the peak plasma concentration is reached in an hour, the peak pharmacological effect does not occur for 48 hours.

e **False** Phenytoin is a hepatic enzyme inducing drug and leads to reduced action of warfarin. Withdrawal of long-term co-administered phenytoin can lead to haemorrhage if the dose of warfarin is not reduced.

Peck T, Hill S, and Williams M (2004) *Pharmacology for Anaesthesia and Intensive Care*, 2nd edition. Cambridge: Cambridge University Press.
Yentis S, Hirsh N, and Smith G (2003) *Anaesthesia and Intensive Care A to Z*, 3rd edition. London: Butterworth-Heinemann.

10 One litre of Gelofusine® contains:

a **False** It is 154 mmol/l.

b **False** It is 125 mmol/l.

c **False** It is 0.4 mmol/l.

d **False** It is 0.4 mmol/l.

e **False** It is 0.4 mmol/l.

Aitkenhead A and Smith G (2008) *Textbook of Anaesthesia*, 5th edition. Edinburgh: Churchill Livingstone.

11 ACE inhibitors:

a **True** They block the conversion of angiotensin I to angiotensin II, which is mediated by ACE and occurs primarily in the pulmonary circulation.

b **False** They are usually administered without diuretics as this can lead to severe hypotension.

c **False** ACE inhibitors cause vasodilation, which may lead to a profound drop in blood pressure, especially with the first dose.

d **True** Angiotensin II acts to constrict renal efferent arterioles and therefore improve perfusion of the glomerulus. ACE inhibitors abolish this and can cause renal impairment, especially in the presence of pre-existing renovascular disease.

e **True** Angioedema is thought to be secondary to a build-up of bradykinins, which are normally metabolized by ACE.

Peck T, Hill S, and Williams M (2004) *Pharmacology for Anaesthesia and Intensive Care*, 2nd edition. Cambridge: Cambridge University Press.

12 Regarding local anaesthetic toxicity:

a **False** The brachial plexus is surrounded by a significant amount of fat in addition to the nerve sheath. Systemic absorption is slower from these areas than from the sacral canal and higher blood levels can be reached after a caudal block.

b **True** Metabolic acidosis, hypoxia, and hypercarbia can all potentiate the negative inotropic effects of local anaesthetic drugs.

c **True** Symptoms such as excitement, tachycardia, and hypertension followed by cardiac irregularities are more associated with esters, and drowsiness, respiratory depression followed by convulsions and circulatory collapse are more commonly associated with amide drugs.

d **False** There is usually a period of CNS excitability leading to convulsions, which occur before cardiovascular effects such as bradycardia, tachyarrhythmias, ventricular fibrillation, and asystole.

e **True** Intralipid® (lipid emulsion) therapy is used alongside standard advanced life support (ALS) measures for the management of cardiac arrest. Resuscitation may need to be prolonged. It may also be useful in treating other lipophilic drug induced cardiac arrests.

Allman K and Wilson I (2006) *Oxford Handbook of Anaesthesia*, 2nd edition. New York: Oxford University Press.

Association of Anaesthetists of Great Britain and Ireland (2007) Guidelines for the management of severe local anaesthetic toxicity. London: Association of Anaesthetists of Great Britain and Ireland. Available at: www.aagbi.org/publications/guidelines.

13 Bicarbonate (HCO_3^-):

a **True** It was a standard therapy in the past but is not used as much now because it can cause intracellular acidosis.

b **False** Bicarbonate is alkaline (pH 8.0) and hypertonic to blood.

c **False** The 8.4% solution contains 84 mg/ml.

d **True** The increase in blood pH moves the curve to the left and therefore impairs delivery of oxygen to the tissues.

e **False** While evidence exists to show improvement in onset times, there are no convincing data on bicarbonate increasing the duration of the block.

Allman K and Wilson I (2006) *Oxford Handbook of Anaesthesia*, 2nd edition. New York: Oxford University Press.

14 One litre of Hartmann's solution contains:

a **False** Na^+ is 131 mmol/l.
b **False** Chloride is 112 mmol/l. Only normal saline has sodium and chloride in equal proportions, i.e. 154 mmol each.
c **True** HCO_3^- is present as lactate.
d **False** K^+ is 5 mmol/l.
e **False** Ca^{2+} is 2 mmol/l.

Aitkenhead A and Smith G (2008) *Textbook of Anaesthesia*, 5th edition. Edinburgh: Churchill Livingstone.

15 Hyoscine:

a **True** Like atropine, it is a natural alkaloid.
b **True** Hyoscine premedication used to be popular for its sedative and antiemetic effects. Caution must be exercised when administering hyoscine to adolescent and elderly patients because it can precipitate delirium.
c **False** Hyoscine is associated with a greater degree of sedation and confusion than atropine.
d **True** Hyoscine reduces sweating and may exacerbate pyrexia; it should be avoided in pyrexial patients, especially children.
e **True** Hyoscine butylbromide (Buscopan) is used regularly in endoscopic procedures and is also used in relieving intestinal colic.

Allman K and Wilson I (2006) *Oxford Handbook of Anaesthesia*, 2nd edition. New York: Oxford University Press.

16 Antifibrinolytic agents include:

a **True** Epsilon-aminocaproic acid was used in ENT surgery. It has been superseded by tranexamic acid and is not available in the UK any more.
b **False** It is an NSAID and indicated for reducing menstrual period pains. It decreases inflammation and contractions of the uterus by inhibition of prostaglandin synthesis.
c **True** Tranexamic acid is 10 times more potent than epsilon-amino caproic acid and is useful in ENT, urology, and vascular surgery among other medical uses.
d **False** It is a fibrinolytic (thrombolytic) drug used in arterial and venous thrombosis and in acute myocardial infarction.
e **True** It is an analogue of vasopressin that causes a twofold to fourfold increase in levels of factor VIII and von Willebrand factor (vWF).

Allman K and Wilson I (2006) *Oxford Handbook of Anaesthesia*, 2nd edition. New York: Oxford University Press.

17 Angiotensin II receptor antagonists:

- a **True** They have the same antihypertensive properties as ACE inhibitors and may cause hyperkalaemia. However, they have fewer systemic side effects such as dry cough and angioedema as they do not affect the breakdown of kinins.
- b **False** ACE inhibitors are known to produce this and consequently many patients have a persistent cough. Angiotensin II antagonists directly inhibit angiotensin II at its smooth muscle receptors, thus avoiding this problem.
- c **False** Angiotensin II receptor antagonists can cause myalgia but have no interaction with muscle relaxant drugs.
- d **False** Hyperkalaemia is more common.
- e **True** The more recent drugs have a half-life of 24 hours.

Peck T, Hill S, and Williams M (2004) *Pharmacology for Anaesthesia and Intensive Care*, 2nd edition. Cambridge: Cambridge University Press.

18 Regarding local anaesthetic drugs:

- a **False** Cocaine was the first local anaesthetic drug to be used. It was used by Karl Koller in 1884 for ophthalmic surgery.
- b **True** Dibucaine, also known as nupercaine and cinchocaine (in the USA), is used for the assay.
- c **True** Prilocaine 2.5% is a constituent of EMLA® topical anaesthetic cream. It may also be used for infiltration and for intravenous regional anaesthesia.
- d **False** The pKa of lidocaine (lignocaine) is 7.9 and the pKa of bupivacaine is 8.1. As the pKa of lidocaine is closer to physiological pH, a larger fraction of the drug is un-ionized and therefore the onset of lidocaine is quicker than that of bupivacaine.
- e **True** This provides useful anaesthesia of the oropharynx, sometimes negating the need for sedation in upper gastrointestinal endoscopy.

Allman K and Wilson I (2006) *Oxford Handbook of Anaesthesia*, 2nd edition. New York: Oxford University Press.

19 NSAIDs:

- a **True** NSAIDs work by inhibition of COX. This leads to a reduction in levels of prostaglandins, prostacyclins, and thromboxanes.
- b **True** Platelet function is reduced by NSAIDs via inhibition of thromboxane production.
- c **False** They reduce the requirement for opiates by 20–40%. They are also used alone to relieve mild to moderate pain.
- d **True** They are more suitable than COX-1 inhibitors. However, one of the COX-2 drugs, rofecoxib has been withdrawn because of concerns of cardiovascular events including myocardial infarction and stroke.
- e **True** They can reduce the glomerular blood flow and exacerbate renal failure.

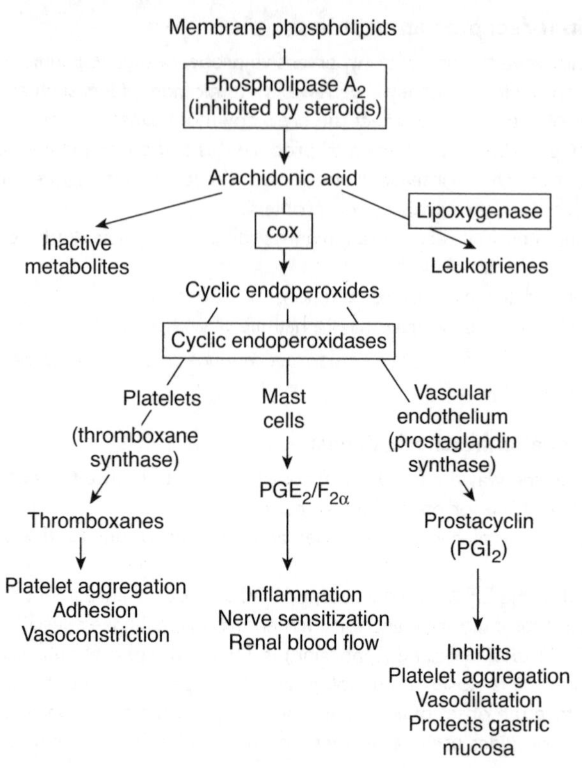

Figure 3.1 Prostaglandin synthesis. COX, cyclo-oxygenase.
Reproduced with kind permission from Kevin K and Spoors C (2009) *Training in Anaesthesia*. New York: Oxford University Press.

Allman K and Wilson I (2006) *Oxford Handbook of Anaesthesia*, 2nd edition. New York: Oxford University Press.

Kevin K and Spoors C (2009) *Training in Anaesthesia*. New York: Oxford University Press.

20 Sugammadex:

a **True** Sugammadex is a modified gamma-cyclodextrin, a selective neuromuscular blocking drug binding agent. It works by encapsulation of the drug and not by interaction with receptors of the neuromuscular junction.

b **False** Sugammadex does not reverse suxamethonium.

c **False** An intubating dose of rocuronium can be reversed within three minutes by administration of sugammadex in an appropriately sufficient dose (16 mg/kg). It is not necessary to wait for any activity to be present on train-of-four monitoring. It is on this basis that rocuronium may eventually replace suxamethonium as the muscle relaxant of choice in rapid sequence induction.

d **False** Sugammadex has been developed for reversal of the aminosteroid neuromuscular blocking drugs, particularly rocuronium, but it will also reverse the action of vecuronium.

e **False** Sugammadex is not contraindicated in diabetes.

Mirakhur RK (2009) Sugammadex in clinical practice. *Anaesthesia* **64** (Suppl. 1):45–54.

21 Metoclopramide:

a **True** It antagonizes dopamine at the chemoreceptor trigger zone.

b **True** It has a good safety and efficacy profile for use in obstetrics and can also be used prior to emergency anaesthesia as its prokinetic action can reduce the gastric residual volume via its cholinergic action, which increases gastric emptying and lowers oesophageal sphincter pressure.

c **False** It increases the lower oesophageal sphincter tone.

d **True** Dopamine inhibitors stimulate release of prolactin. Metoclopramide can cause galactorrhoea and disorders of menstruation.

e **True** Metoclopramide may cause extrapyramidal side effects and acute dystonic reactions, especially when given to children and young adults.

Allman K and Wilson I (2006) *Oxford Handbook of Anaesthesia*, 2nd edition. New York: Oxford University Press.

22 Concerning cholinesterase and anticholinesterases:

a **True** Acetylcholinesterase is found within the basement membrane of the postsynaptic cleft and also within red blood cells and the placenta.

b **True** Pseudo cholinesterase and butyryl cholinesterase are also synonyms.

c **True** Neostigmine is a medium acting drug. Its duration of action is 1 hour after IV and two to four hours after oral administration.

d **True** Ecothiopate eye drops are used in the management of glaucoma. Ecothiopate can reduce the level of plasma cholinesterase and therefore prolong the duration of action of suxamethonium.

e **False** Organophosphorous compounds inhibit the action of acetylcholinesterase by forming a stable complex.

Allman K and Wilson I (2006) *Oxford Handbook of Anaesthesia*, 2nd edition. New York: Oxford University Press.

Yentis S, Hirsh N, and Smith G (2003) *Anaesthesia and Intensive Care A to Z*, 3rd edition. London: Butterworth-Heinemann.

23 Low molecular weight heparins (LMWHs):

a **True** LMWHs enhance the formation of the 'antithrombin III–thrombin' complex and also inhibit factor Xa.

b **False** LMWHs are more effective at inhibiting factor Xa, than forming the antithrombin III–thrombin complex.

c **True** Only a single daily dose is required.

d **False** LMWH is mainly excreted through the kidneys. There is a requirement to reduce the dose in chronic renal failure.

e **False** They do not prolong the APTT as their main effect is factor Xa inhibition. The effect of a standard dose is sufficiently predictable so that monitoring is not required routinely.

Peck T, Hill S, and Williams M (2004) *Pharmacology for Anaesthesia and Intensive Care*, 2nd edition. Cambridge: Cambridge University Press.

24 Protamine:

a **True** Protamine is a protein extracted from fish sperm including salmon.

b **True** Protamine is basic and heparin is acidic. Protamine undergoes a chemical reaction in the presence of heparin and forms an inactive complex, thus neutralizing the action of heparin.

c **True** Severe anaphylactic reactions are associated with protamine which can be lethal. There is a suggestion that vasectomized men develop antibodies to sperm and are therefore at risk of an allergic reaction when subsequently exposed to protamine. Patients taking insulin prepared with protamine may also experience reactions.

d **False** Protamine is associated with myocardial depression and hypotension, and for this reason must be administered slowly to reduce these effects.

e **True** Protamine has a weak anticoagulant action on its own and can promote bleeding if given far in excess of the dose required to neutralize heparin.

Peck T, Hill S, and Williams M (2004) *Pharmacology for Anaesthesia and Intensive Care*, 2nd edition. Cambridge: Cambridge University Press.

25 Cisatracurium:

a **True** Cisatracurium is one of the isomers of atracurium.

b **False** Cis-atracurium is medium acting, with effects lasting approximately 40–55 minutes.

c **False** Metabolic acidosis seems to prolong its action compared with atracurium, whose duration of action reduces in the presence of acidosis.

d **False** It is around 0.15 mg/kg for intubation and 0.03 mg/kg for maintenance.

e **True** Cisatracurium causes minimal release of histamine compared with atracurium.

Allman K and Wilson I (2006) *Oxford Handbook of Anaesthesia*, 2nd edition. New York: Oxford University Press.

26 Vecuronium:

a **True** It is a mono-quaternary aminosteroid, structurally similar to pancuronium.

b **False** Its average duration of action is 30–40 minutes.

c **False** Unlike pancuronium, vecuronium does not have any action on heart rate.

d **False** Vecuronium is only 20% metabolized, 70% is excreted in bile and 30% in urine.

e **True** Vecuronium is metabolized to 3- and 17-hydroxy and 3,17 dihydroxyvecuronium. The 3-hydroxy vecuronium possesses muscle-relaxant properties which may accumulate during administration as an infusion and can prolong the action of the drug.

Peck T, Hill S, and Williams M (2004) *Pharmacology for Anaesthesia and Intensive Care*, 2nd edition. Cambridge: Cambridge University Press.
Rang H, Dale M, and Ritter J (2000) *Rang and Dales' Pharmacology*, 6th edition. Edinburgh: Churchill Livingstone.

27 Metaraminol:

a **False** Metaraminol is a directly and indirectly acting sympathomimetic drug. It has predominantly alpha 1 adrenoceptor action but also some beta activity.
b **False** It is associated with hypertension and reflex bradycardia.
c **False** The duration of action is approximately 20–30 minutes.
d **True** It can decrease renal and placental blood flow and for this reason is avoided in the treatment of hypotension caused by regional anaesthesia in obstetric practice.
e **True** It should be avoided in patients with hyperthyroidism and those taking MAOIs as it may be associated with excessive hypertension.

Allman K and Wilson I (2006) *Oxford Handbook of Anaesthesia*, 2nd edition. New York: Oxford University Press.

28 Phentolamine:

a **True** Phentolamine is a competitive non-selective alpha blocker.
b **True** It is used for the treatment of excessive hypertensive events such as in MAOI reactions and phaeochromocytoma manipulation.
c **False** The alpha blockade causes vasodilation and there is reflex tachycardia, which maintains the cardiac output.
d **True** Vasodilation of the vessels of the nasal mucosa leads to nasal congestion.
e **False** Noradrenaline (norepinephrine) or methoxamine should be used in this situation because adrenaline (epinephrine) has strong beta effects which increase the tachycardia further.

Allman K and Wilson I (2006) *Oxford Handbook of Anaesthesia*, 2nd edition. New York: Oxford University Press.

29 Amethocaine:

a **True** Amethocaine is also known as tetracaine.
b **True** The name Ametop® is derived from 'amethocaine topical'.
c **False** Amethocaine is an ester and as such is associated with more cutaneous irritation than the amide topical local anaesthetics. The first amide local anaesthetic drug, lidocaine (lignocaine) was synthesized in 1943 but was not used clinically until 1948.
d **False** It is prilocaine, a constituent of EMLA®, which is associated with methaemoglobinaemia.
e **True** The duration of action of topical amethocaine eye drops is long, up to four hours.

Allman K and Wilson I (2006) *Oxford Handbook of Anaesthesia*, 2nd edition. New York: Oxford University Press.

30 Drugs to be avoided in asthma include:

a **False** Etomidate is considered safe for induction.
b **False** Although histamine release is significant with the use of suxamethonium, it has not been found to be unsafe in asthma.
c **False** It is one of the most potent bronchodilators among all of the IV induction agents. Despite its CNS effects it is a very useful induction agent in severe asthma.
d **False** Rocuronium has not been associated with bronchospasm, in contrast with atracurium, which is associated with significant histamine release.
e **False** Pethidine has an atropine-like action and hence is safer than morphine in this situation.

Allman K and Wilson I (2006) *Oxford Handbook of Anaesthesia*, 2nd edition. New York: Oxford University Press.

chapter 3 PHYSICS

QUESTIONS

1 The expiratory valve in a breathing circuit:

a Is known as an active pressure levered valve
b Is also known as the spill or relief valve
c Opens during expiration at a pressure of approximately 3 cmH_2O
d Has a pressure relief safety mechanism when it is completely closed for invasive positive pressure ventilation (IPPV) and is actuated at a pressure of 40 cmH_2O
e May remain continuously open during respiration if there is a malfunction in the scavenging system attached to it

2 Essential monitoring for anaesthesia includes:

a Capnography
b BIS
c Temperature
d Vapour analysis
e Airway pressure

3 The pulse oximeter:

a Monitors the oxygen saturation continuously
b Is accurate between 60% and 100% saturation
c Averages its readings every 10–20 seconds
d Response time to desaturation is approximately 60 seconds using an ear probe and 10–15 seconds using the finger probe
e May give inaccurate results if applied to an area with high venous pulsation

4 A breathing circuit reservoir bag:

a When used with a T-piece (Mapleson F) is double ended
b Is made of antistatic rubber or plastic
c Has a 1 litre capacity in paediatric circuits
d Has 3 litres capacity in adult circuits
e Is an accurate guide of the patient's tidal volume

5 Information displayed on a medical cylinder label includes:

a The cylinder size code
b Filling date, shelf-life, and expiratory date
c Substance identification number and batch number
d Filling ratio
e The date of the last cylinder testing

6 Regarding the vacuum-insulated evaporator (VIE):

a It contains liquid oxygen
b The temperature in the VIE is maintained at −118°C
c The pressure within the VIE is 700 kPa
d A safety valve opens at 900 kPa, allowing oxygen to escape if there is excess pressure in the VIE
e It can produce 842 times its volume as gas at 15°C

7 Concerning oxygen concentrators:

a They extract oxygen from air by differential absorption
b A single zeolite molecular sieve is used to filter the air
c Filtered air is pressurized to about 170 kPa using a compressor
d A maximum oxygen concentration of 90% is achieved
e The non-oxygen fraction left over is composed of nitrogen and helium

8 Entonox®:

a Is a 50:50 mixture of nitrous oxide and oxygen by weight
b Is delivered by a self-administered, continuous flow system
c Cylinders show the same gauge pressure as oxygen cylinders when full
d Cylinders are preferably stored in the horizontal position when ambient temperature is low
e Is a safe method of analgesia for a patient with a pneumothorax

9 Concerning pressure gauges:

a The Bourdon gauge is an example
b They utilize a tube which uncoils, attached to a pointer on a display
c Each gauge is gas-specific
d The pressure gauge accurately reflects the remaining contents of both oxygen and nitrous oxide cylinders
e The gauges for pipeline and cylinder pressure measurement are interchangeable

10 Piped medical gas supply:

a Is supplied from a bank of cylinders or from an oxygen tank
b Is delivered by bronze alloy, bacteriostatic pipes
c Hoses are attached to the anaesthetic machine via a universal connector
d The gas outlets are colour and shape coded
e The tug test is performed to detect misconnection

11 Pressure regulators:

a Are reducing valves
b Use a spring and diaphragm mechanism
c Reduce cylinder pressure to 700 kPa as it enters the back bar of the anaesthetic machine
d Protect the patient from sudden surges of pressure from the cylinders
e Have a relief valve downstream, opening at a pressure of 1000 kPa

12 Flow meters:

- a Have a flow control or needle valve at the base to regulate gas flow
- b Increase gas flow when the control knob is turned clockwise
- c Are calibrated in 2 litre graduations
- d Are fitted with interactive oxygen and nitrous oxide controls to prevent delivery of a hypoxic mixture
- e They are accurate to within 1% of the flow rate

13 Vaporizers:

- a Deliver a precise concentration of inhalational agent despite changes in fresh gas flow during use
- b With 'Tec' attached to the name indicates that it is a temperature controlled or compensated device
- c Must be recalibrated for use at high altitude
- d Of the Plenum variety have a low internal resistance to gas flow
- e Of Tec Mark 4 type have a temperature-sensitive valve within the vaporizing chamber

14 Three-lead electrocardiogram (ECG) recording:

- a Measures the electrical activity of the heart with electrical potentials of 2–3 mV
- b Is useful in determining heart rate and arrhythmias and accurately assessing signs of ischaemia
- c Uses skin electrodes made of silver/silver chloride
- d In the CM5 configuration, the right arm lead is placed over the manubrium, the left arm lead is over the mid-axillary line in fifth intercostal space and the indifferent lead is over the left shoulder
- e Can lead to burns from the ECG electrodes if the diathermy plate is incorrectly positioned.

15 Sources of error in pulse oximetry include:

- a Carboxyhaemoglobin giving a false high reading
- b Methaemoglobin giving a false low reading
- c HbF giving a low reading
- d Bilirubin giving a low reading
- e Methylene blue giving a false low reading

16 Endotracheal tubes:

- a Are made from polyvinyl chloride if they are single use
- b Have the outer diameter marked in millimetres, on the outside
- c Have a right facing bevel in order to facilitate ventilation to the right lung, if the tube is advanced too far
- d Have a black intubation depth marker 5 cm proximal to the cuff in some designs
- e May have 'IT' marked on them to indicate that they have been implantation tested

17 Concerning capnography:

- a End-tidal carbon dioxide is equal to arterial carbon dioxide
- b The infrared absorption principle is used in capnography
- c A photo-acoustic technique can also be used for estimation of carbon dioxide
- d A waveform that does not return to baseline during inspiration can indicate a faulty Mapleson D breathing system.
- e A sloping plateau of the waveform is seen in patients with chronic obstructive pulmonary disease

18 Anaesthetic face masks:

- a Are made of silicone rubber or plastic
- b Can be used with an anaesthetic circuit to deliver 100% oxygen
- c Can increase the dead space by up to 50 ml in adults
- d Can cause nerve palsies during prolonged use
- e Are available to cover the nose only for use in dental chair anaesthesia

19 Concerning laryngoscopes:

- a The Macintosh laryngoscope is designed to lift the epiglottis
- b Straight blade laryngoscopes cause more vagal stimulation than the curved blades
- c A polio blade is useful in patients with a short neck
- d The McCoy laryngoscope is available both as a curved and straight blade
- e Disposable laryngoscopy equipment must be used for tonsillectomy patients

20 Medical gas cylinders:

- a Are made from lightweight molybdenum steel
- b At constant temperature, a half-empty oxygen cylinder will display the same pressure as a full cylinder, i.e. 13 700 kPa
- c Are available in sizes A to M
- d Of E size are used on the anaesthetic machine
- e Of J size are commonly used for cylinder manifolds

21 The circle breathing system:

- a Is suitable for paediatric or adult use
- b Is one of the ways of reducing pollution in theatre
- c Can be used for low flow anaesthesia for economy
- d Does not require any priming before use for low flow anaesthesia
- e May produce carbon monoxide with dry soda-lime

22 The Humphrey breathing system:

- a Is a combined Mapleson ADE system
- b Can be used safely in adults and children
- c Requires a fresh gas flow of 70–100 ml/kg for spontaneous ventilation in adults
- d Requires a minimum of 5 l/min flow for children below 25 kg
- e Is not suitable for controlled ventilation

23 Colour coding of gas cylinders is as follows:

a	Oxygen	Black body with white shoulders
b	Oxygen/helium	Black with grey and white shoulder quarters
c	Air	Grey with white and black shoulder quarters
d	Carbon dioxide	Grey with grey shoulders
e	Nitrous oxide	Blue with white and blue quarters

24 Heat and moisture exchange (HME) humidifiers:

a Are able to provide 75–85% relative humidity
b Warm the inspired gases to between 35°C and 40°C
c Require five to 20 minutes before they reach the optimal ability to humidify dry gases
d May add approximately 25 ml of dead space when used in adults
e Can be converted to heat and moisture exchange filters (HMEF) by having a pore size of 0.5 μm to filter out bacteria.

25 Concerning temperature

a The intervals on the Celsius and Kelvin scales are identical
b The Kelvin is equal to 1/273.16 of the triple point of water
c The triple point of water occurs at 0.1°C
d The triple point of water is the temperature when water vapour and liquid are in equal concentrations
e The temperature of a gas is a measure of the speed of movement of its molecules

26 Regarding temperature measurement:

a In the electrical resistance thermometer, the electrical resistance is inversely proportional to the temperature
b The thermistor utilizes the Seebeck effect
c The thermocouple relies on production of voltage where two dissimilar metals join
d Mercury thermometers are suitable for reading very low temperatures
e A thermistor contains a semiconducting metal with a resistance that increases as temperature increases

27 The classic laryngeal mask airway (LMA™):

a Is made of silicone rubber
b Can be used a maximum of 50 times
c Is not suitable for use in the magnetic resonance imaging (MRI) scanner
d Has an internal diameter of 8, 12, 12, and 14 mm for sizes 2, 3, 4, and 5, respectively
e Is strengthened by a stainless steel wire spiral in the reinforced version

28 The Clark electrode:

a Is used for measuring oxygen saturation in the blood
b Is also known as a polarographic oxygen analyser
c Has a faster response time than the fuel cell
d Can measure oxygen in a sample of gas
e Is robust and has a life expectancy of five years

29 Concerning cylinder valves:

a They are made of copper alloy and screwed into the neck of the cylinder via a threaded connection

b They have the chemical formula of the gas in the cylinder engraved the side

c The non-interchangeable pin index position for oxygen is 3 and 5 and for nitrous oxide is 2 and 5

d A safety relief device allows the discharge of cylinder contents to the atmosphere if the cylinder is over-pressurized

e A compressible yoke sealing washer must be placed between the valve outlet and the apparatus to make a gas-tight connection

30 Methods of non-invasive blood pressure monitoring include:

a Palpation

b The Riva–Rocci method

c Oscillotonometry

d The oscillometric method

e The plethysmographic method

chapter 3

PHYSICS

ANSWERS

1 The expiratory valve in a breathing circuit:

a **False** It is known as an adjustable pressure limiting (APL) valve.

b **True** It does not allow room air to enter the breathing system, allowing only expiration through it.

c **False** During spontaneous ventilation, a pressure of less than 1 cmH_2O or 0.1 kPa is needed to actuate it when it is in the open position.

d **False** During assisted ventilation, the APL opens at 60 cmH_2O in the closed position to avoid exposing the patient to excessive pressures.

e **True** If excessive negative pressure is applied to the expiratory vent by a malfunctioning scavenging system the valve may remain open, leading to a large increase in dead space.

Al-Shaikh B and Stacey S (2006) *Essentials of Anaesthetic Equipment*, 3rd edition. Edinburgh: Churchill Livingstone.

2 Essential monitoring for anaesthesia includes:

a **True** Capnography provides information not only on the respiratory and cardiovascular status of the patient but also gives early warning of disconnection of the breathing system.

b **False** At present it is not essential to have sophisticated monitors of depth of anaesthesia, for example bispectral index (BIS). It is essential, however, that the anaesthetist be present throughout to monitor the patient clinically.

c **False** Although temperature measurement is important, especially since the introduction of the National Institute for Health and Clinical Excellence (NICE) guidelines on inadvertent perioperative hypothermia, thermometers are not essential monitors but must be available.

d **True** Monitoring of the patient's airway gases, oxygen, carbon dioxide, and inhalational anaesthetic agents, if used, is essential.

e **True** When IPPV is used, airway pressure alarms must also be enabled and set to appropriate limits.

Association of Anaesthetists of Great Britain and Ireland (2007) *Recommendations for Standards of Monitoring during Anaesthesia and Recovery*, 4th edition. London: Association of Anaesthetists of Great Britain and Ireland.

3 The pulse oximeter:

a **True** The high frequency LEDs allow absorption to be sampled many times during each pulse beat. Running averages of saturation are calculated many times per second.
b **False** As the pulse oximeter is calibrated from healthy volunteers it is accurate between 70% and 100%, as this was the range used in the experiments. Below 70% the readings are extrapolated.
c **True** Because the readings are averaged oximeters cannot detect acute desaturation, as there is a time delay of up to 60 seconds depending on the site of the probe.
d **False** The ear probe is more sensitive than the finger probe and has a response time of 10–15 seconds. The finger probe may take 60 seconds or more to respond to desaturation.
e **True** The pulse oximeter works on the assumption that any pulsatile absorption is caused by arterial pulsation only.

Al-Shaikh B and Stacey S (2006) *Essentials of Anaesthetic Equipment*, 3rd edition. Edinburgh: Churchill Livingstone.

4 A breathing circuit reservoir bag:

a **True** When the bag is used as part of a T-piece system the bag has an opening at both ends, the smaller end acts as an expiratory port. It can be partially occluded to provide continuous positive airway pressure (CPAP) or positive end-expiratory pressure (PEEP).
b **True** It is also latex free.
c **False** The paediatric bag usually is 0.5 litres in capacity.
d **False** The standard adult bag size is 2 litres. If the bag is too large it does not provide a reliable monitor of respiration in spontaneously ventilating patients.
e **False** Although it is a good indicator of respiratory efforts and pattern, it is only an inaccurate guide of tidal volume.

Al-Shaikh B and Stacey S (2006) *Essentials of Anaesthetic Equipment*, 3rd edition. Edinburgh: Churchill Livingstone.

5 Information displayed on a medical cylinder label includes:

a **True** Each cylinder used clinically has its size marked on the label. Sizes A and H are not used for medical gases.
b **True** This information is useful for storage and rotation of cylinders in use.
c **True** The batch number of a cylinder is an important piece of information in the event of any clinical problems during use. Cylinders from that batch can be isolated and sent for analysis rather than sending all the cylinders back to the manufacturer. Prior to batch labelling, a situation had occurred where contaminated nitrous oxide cylinders caused two cases of pulmonary oedema, one of which was fatal (reported by Clutton-Brock, 1967). Since there was no clear information on the cylinders, all nitrous oxide cylinders were withdrawn from use throughout Britain.
d **False** The filling ratio is the weight of fluid in the cylinder divided by the weight of water required to fill the cylinder. This is not displayed on the label. The filling ratio for nitrous oxide it is 0.75 in the UK and 0.67 in hotter climates, to prevent dangerous increase in pressure with raised temperature.
e **False** This is identified by the shape and the colour of a plastic disc around the neck of the cylinder.

Al-Shaikh B and Stacey S (2006) *Essentials of Anaesthetic Equipment*, 3rd edition. Edinburgh: Churchill Livingstone.
Clutton-Brock J (1967) Two cases of poisoning by contamination of nitrous oxide with higher oxides of nitrogen during anaesthesia. *Br J Anaesth* **39**:388.

6 Regarding the vacuum-insulated evaporator (VIE):

- a **True** It is the most economical way of storing oxygen.
- b **False** The critical temperature of oxygen is –118°C. The temperature within the VIE is below this, at –150 to –170°C.
- c **True** The pressure within the VIE is 7 bar (700 kPa). A pressure regulator then reduces the pressure to pipeline pressure of 4.1 bar (410 kPa).
- d **False** The safety valve opens at a pressure of 1700 kPa when there is a build up of pressure within the VIE, which can be caused by under-demand for oxygen.
- e **True** This explains why it is an efficient way of storing oxygen.

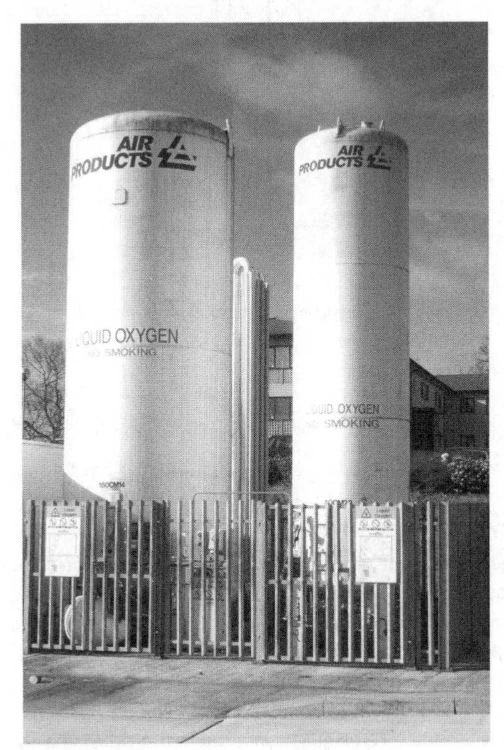

Figure 3.2 A vacuum-insulated evaporator.
Reproduced with kind permission from Kevin K and Spoors C (2009) *Training in Anaesthesia*. New York: Oxford University Press.

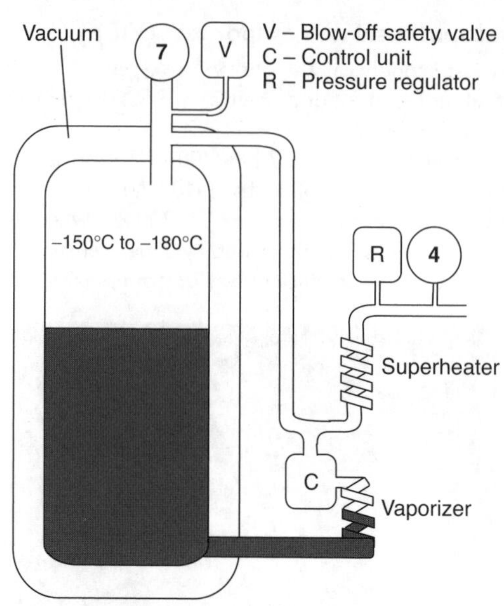

Figure 3.3 Schematic diagram of the inside of a vacuum-insulated evaporator.
Reproduced with kind permission from Kevin K and Spoors C (2009) *Training in Anaesthesia*. New York: Oxford University Press.

Al-Shaikh B and Stacey S (2006) *Essentials of Anaesthetic Equipment*, 3rd edition. Edinburgh: Churchill Livingstone.
Kevin K and Spoors C (2009) *Training in Anaesthesia*. New York: Oxford University Press.

7 Concerning oxygen concentrators:

a **True** Nitrogen and other unwanted components of air are retained and then vented into the atmosphere after heating and applying a vacuum.
b **False** Many zeolite columns are used for this process and the columns used are changed over periodically.
c **False** The filtered air is pressurized to 137 kPa.
d **False** The maximum concentration is 95% by volume.
e **False** Argon is the main remaining constituent, the others having been released to the atmosphere already.

Al-Shaikh B and Stacey S (2006) *Essentials of Anaesthetic Equipment*, 3rd edition. Edinburgh: Churchill Livingstone.

8 Entonox®:

a **False** It is a 50:50 mixture of oxygen and nitrous oxide by volume.

b **False** It is self-administered through a demand flow system.

c **True** The gauge pressure on a cylinder of Entonox® is 13 700 kPa or 137 bar. A high pressure is required to maintain both components in gaseous form.

d **True** If the temperature drops below –5.5°C liquefaction and separation of nitrous oxide and oxygen can occur. This process can be prevented by storing the cylinders horizontally to ensure mixing and an adequate area for diffusion to occur. Cylinders should be stored above 5°C before use to prevent a hypoxic mixture being delivered to the patient.

e **False** The nitrous oxide expands in air-filled cavities as it diffuses in more rapidly than nitrogen diffuses out. It should therefore not be used in a patient with a pneumothorax as it can expand and tension.

Aitkenhead A and Smith G. (2008) *Textbook of Anaesthesia*, 5th edition. Edinburgh: Churchill Livingstone.

Al-Shaikh B and Stacey S (2006) *Essentials of Anaesthetic Equipment*, 3rd edition. Edinburgh: Churchill Livingstone.

9 Pressure gauges:

a **True** The Bourdon gauge is one of the earliest designs in use.

b **True** The coiled tube is subjected to the pressure within the gas cylinder. When the tube uncoils, it moves the needle pointer over a dial indicating pressure.

c **True** Each gauge is calibrated for a particular gas.

d **False** It is applicable only to oxygen, which is stored as a gas, and therefore the pressure inside the cylinder will reflect the state of emptying of the cylinder. Nitrous oxide is stored as a liquid and vapour and does not behave like a perfect gas that follows Boyle's law (pressure × volume = constant).

e **False** The gauges designed for use on pipelines should not be used to measure gas cylinder pressure and vice versa. This is to prevent damage and inaccurate measurement.

Al-Shaikh B and Stacey S (2006) *Essentials of Anaesthetic Equipment*, 3rd edition. Edinburgh: Churchill Livingstone.

10 Piped medical gas supply:

a **True** It is delivered at a pressure of 400 kPa. Special outlet valves supply various parts of the hospital.

b **False** The pipeline is made of high quality copper alloy which prevents degradation of the gases and has bacteriostatic properties.

c **False** Each pipeline is permanently attached to the anaesthetic machine end via a non-interchangeable screw thread (NIST) nut and liner. Each thread has a unique pattern so the wrong pipeline cannot be attached to the anaesthetic machine.

d **True** Each gas outlet is colour and shape coded and each hose has an index collar and locking groove so that each hose can only fit into its correct supply outlet to avoid cross connection.

e **True** If the hose is not properly locked into the supply outlet it will come out when tugged. The test in itself may wear the connections.

Al-Shaikh B and Stacey S (2006) *Essentials of Anaesthetic Equipment*, 3rd edition. Edinburgh: Churchill Livingstone.

11 Pressure regulators:

a **True** The pressure regulator is positioned between the cylinder and the anaesthetic machine and converts the higher variable pressure in the gas cylinder to a constant lower pressure.

b **True** The gas from a high pressure chamber enters the low pressure chamber via a valve. The high pressure tries to close the valve but the opposing force of the diaphragm and spring does the opposite. Thus a balance is reached between the two opposing forces, maintaining gas flow at a constant pressure of 400 kPa.

c **False** The pressure is reduced from that within the cylinder, 13 700 kPa for oxygen, to its operating pressure of 400 kPa as it enters the anaesthetic machine.

d **False** They protect the anaesthetic machine from pressure surges.

e **False** The pressure relief valve is usually set to 700 kPa and thus allow escape of gas if the pressure regulators fail, avoiding damage to the anaesthetic machine.

Al-Shaikh B and Stacey S (2006) *Essentials of Anaesthetic Equipment*, 3rd edition. Edinburgh: Churchill Livingstone.

12 Flow meters:

a **True** Flow control valves allow manual adjustment of gas flow.

b **False** Rotation of the control knob anticlockwise increases the gas flow rate.

c **False** Above the 1 litre mark they are calibrated in litres/min. Below the 1 litre mark the calibrations are in 100 ml/min. Some anaesthetic machines have an additional flow meter measuring up to 1 litre/min maximum in series with the standard flow meter. This allows fine control during low flow anaesthesia.

d **True** Accidental reduction in oxygen flow reduces the nitrous oxide flow while preventing the oxygen from shutting off completely.

e **False** They have an accuracy of approximately 2.5%.

Al-Shaikh B and Stacey S (2006) *Essentials of Anaesthetic Equipment*, 3rd edition. Edinburgh: Churchill Livingstone.

13 Vaporizers:

a **True** The modern design of vaporizers allows them to be able to deliver a precise concentration of inhalational agent even with flows ranging from 0.5 litres to 15 litres per minute.

b **True** The 'Tec' indicates temperature compensation for the changes in temperature which occur with the loss of latent heat of vaporization as the volatile becomes vapour. Temperature compensation is via a heat sink and the use of a bimetallic strip which alters the amount of fresh gas flow entering the vaporizing chamber.

c **False** The product of partial pressure and the saturated vapour pressure remains the same and therefore no recalibration is required at high altitudes.

d **False** Plenum vaporizers have high internal resistance whereas the draw-over vaporizers have low internal resistance to gas flow.

e **False** Tec Mark 3, 4, and 5 vaporizers all have the temperature-sensitive valve, which controls the splitting ratio situated outside the vaporizing chamber. The Mark 2 vaporizer has the valve within the vaporizing chamber.

Al-Shaikh B and Stacey S (2006) *Essentials of Anaesthetic Equipment*, 3rd edition. Edinburgh: Churchill Livingstone.

14 Three-lead electrocardiogram (ECG) recording:

a **False** Electrical potentials between 0.5 and 2 mV at the skin surface are measured.

b **False** Although a reasonable assumption of ischaemia can be made, a full 12-lead ECG is required to provide a clear picture of myocardial ischaemia.

c **True** Silver/silver chloride forms a stable electrode combination. Both are held in a cup and separated from the skin by a foam pad soaked in conducting gel.

d **False** The CM5 configuration is able to detect 89% of ST segment changes due to left ventricular ischaemia. Hence positioning of electrodes is of vital importance. The right arm lead is placed over the manubrium, the left arm lead is in the fifth intercostal space in the left anterior axillary line, and the indifferent lead is over the left shoulder or any other point.

e **True** Passage of diathermy current via the electrodes may cause a high current density and therefore damage to the tissue underneath.

Al-Shaikh B and Stacey S (2006) *Essentials of Anaesthetic Equipment*, 3rd edition. Edinburgh: Churchill Livingstone.

15 Sources of error in pulse oximetry include:

a **True** A falsely high reading is seen with carbon monoxide poisoning where there is an increased level of carboxyhaemoglobin.

b **True** In the presence of methaemoglobin the oximeter tends to read lower in the range of 85%.

c **False** The absorption spectrum is similar to adult haemoglobin over the range of wave lengths used.

d **False** Bilirubin does not have any effect on saturation reading.

e **True** In the same way indocyanine green used in cardiac output measurement can give a false low reading in the 80% range.

Al-Shaikh B and Stacey S (2006) *Essentials of Anaesthetic Equipment*, 3rd edition. Edinburgh: Churchill Livingstone.

16 Endotracheal tubes:

a **True** PVC tubes are non-irritant to the airway and can be used safely for longer periods of ventilation. Red rubber tubes although still available in a few places cannot be used for prolonged ventilation.

b **False** The internal diameter is marked in millimetres on the tube.

c **False** Most tube designs have a left facing bevel and some have an additional side hole opposite the bevel, called Murphy's eye. This facilitates ventilation in the event of a blockage from secretions, blood, or the wall of the trachea.

d **False** The intubation marker is 3 cm proximal to the cuff.

e **True** The original Portex tubes had 'IT' marked on them to indicate implantation testing. A small quantity of the plastic mould was implanted under the skin of a rabbit and observed for any signs of irritation or inflammation. If no irritation occurred that batch was sent for production.

Al-Shaikh B and Stacey S (2006) *Essentials of Anaesthetic Equipment*, 3rd edition. Edinburgh: Churchill Livingstone.

17 Concerning capnography:

a **False** End-tidal carbon dioxide is 0.3–0.6 kPa lower than arterial levels.
b **True** The difference in the absorption of infrared light between the sample gas and the reference gas is the basis of the estimation.
c **True** In these devices the sample gas is irradiated with infrared light of a suitable wavelength. The periodic expansion and contraction produces a pressure fluctuation of audible frequency that can be detected with a microphone. This method is much more accurate although it is not used in clinical practice.
d **True** A trace that does not return to baseline indicates rebreathing is occurring. This could be due to exhaustion of soda-lime, a faulty breathing system, or extreme tachypnoea.
e **True** The waveform shows a sloping trace and does not accurately reflect the end-tidal carbon dioxide.

Al-Shaikh B and Stacey S (2006) *Essentials of Anaesthetic Equipment*, 3rd edition. Edinburgh: Churchill Livingstone.

18 Anaesthetic face masks:

a **True** The masks used in the past were opaque black. The transparent masks in use currently enable closer monitoring of patients, e.g. by misting of the mask or the presence of blood, secretions, or vomit.
b **True** An efficient method of delivering 100% oxygen non-invasively is through a well-fitting face mask and an anaesthetic breathing circuit.
c **False** The dead space of an adult mask could be as much as 200 ml.
d **True** Especially when used with a tight fitting facial harness nerve palsies have been reported, e.g. facial nerve palsy.
e **True** Nasal masks are available for use in dental chair anaesthesia.

Al-Shaikh B and Stacey S (2006) *Essentials of Anaesthetic Equipment*, 3rd edition. Edinburgh: Churchill Livingstone.

19 Concerning laryngoscopes:

a **True** The Macintosh laryngoscope is passed along the tongue up to the vallecula. The upward lift from this position actually lifts the larynx by the stretching of aryepiglottic ligaments.
b **True** Straight-bladed laryngoscopes are passed beyond the tip of the epiglottis and stimulate the posterior surface of the epiglottis as it is lifted to view the larynx. Since this surface is innervated by the internal laryngeal branch of the superior laryngeal nerve, a branch of the vagus, bradycardia is more likely, especially during emergency intubation in the presence of hypoxia and hypercarbia.
c **True** The polio blade was originally designed to intubate patients ventilated in the iron lung. The blade is at about 120° to the handle allowing easier laryngoscopy. It is very useful in patients with large breasts, and may be of use in short-necked individuals as well.
d **True** The McCoy laryngoscope was designed as a curved blade originally, but is now available as a straight blade as well.
e **True** Due to concerns over variant Creutzfeldt–Jakob disease (vCJD), patients undergoing tonsillectomy must have disposable airway equipment. Most laryngoscope blades are single use; if a reusable blade is used, it must be covered with a plastic sheath. Single-use supraglottic airway devices are also available in standard and reinforced designs.

Al-Shaikh B and Stacey S (2006) *Essentials of Anaesthetic Equipment*, 3rd edition. Edinburgh: Churchill Livingstone.

20 Medical gas cylinders:

- a **True** They are designed to withstand considerable internal pressure.
- b **False** Since oxygen is a gas it obeys Boyle's law, and therefore the pressure in a half-empty cylinder will be half of 13 700 kPa, i.e. 6850 kPa.
- c **False** They are available in sizes A to L. The most commonly used sizes in the hospital are D, E, and F.
- d **True** An E cylinder contains 680 litres of oxygen and is the one commonly attached to the anaesthetic machine.
- e **True** A number of J cylinders may be used as a cylinder manifold to supply smaller hospitals as an alternative to supply from a VIE.

Al-Shaikh B and Stacey S (2006) *Essentials of Anaesthetic Equipment*, 3rd edition. Edinburgh: Churchill Livingstone.
BOC Medical. Medical gas cylinder data chart. Available at: www.bocmedical.co.uk.

21 The circle breathing system:

- a **True** During paediatric use a smaller soda-lime canister may be required. Some increase in resistance to respiration is to be expected during spontaneous respiration and close monitoring is essential.
- b **True** The lower fresh gas flow (FGF) used leads to a reduction in theatre pollution.
- c **True** A FGF of less than 1.5 litres/min is adequate in an adult and this amounts to a considerable cost saving.
- d **False** High FGF for several minutes is required to de-nitrogenate the circle system and the functional residual capacity (FRC) of the patient, to prevent a build-up of nitrogen in the circuit. In closed circle system anaesthesia a high FGF is needed for up to 15 minutes at the beginning of anaesthesia.
- e **True** When inhalational agents with the CHF_2 moiety such as enflurane or isoflurane are used carbon monoxide may form especially when the soda lime is totally dry. Newer soda-lime is supposed to be free from this problem.

Al-Shaikh B and Stacey S (2006) *Essentials of Anaesthetic Equipment*, 3rd edition. Edinburgh: Churchill Livingstone.

22 The Humphrey breathing system:

- a **True** It is also known as the Humphrey ADE system.
- b **True** As the name implies an E circuit is incorporated in the system for use in paediatrics.
- c **False** A FGF of 50–60 ml/kg/min is more than adequate in adults.
- d **False** A FGF of 3 l/min in children less than 25 kg in weight is safe
- e **False** It is a versatile system and allows spontaneous and controlled ventilation in both children and adults.

Al-Shaikh B and Stacey S (2006) *Essentials of Anaesthetic Equipment*, 3rd edition. Edinburgh: Churchill Livingstone.

23 Colour coding of gas cylinders is as follows:

- a **True** In the USA, oxygen cylinders are green.
- b **False** It has a black body with white/brown quarters on the shoulder.
- c **True** In the USA, air is contained in yellow cylinders.
- d **True** Although carbon dioxide is no longer mounted on the anaesthetic machines, it is used for laparoscopic procedures.
- e **False** Nitrous oxide cylinder is uniformly blue on the body and shoulder. A cylinder that has a blue body and white and blue quarters on the shoulder contains Entonox®.

Table 3.2 The characteristics of different cylinders

	Body colour	Shoulder colour	Contains	Pressure when full (bar)*	Pin index
Oxygen	Black	White	Gas	137	2,5
Nitrous oxide	Blue	Blue	Liquid and vapour	45	3,5
Entonox®	Blue	White/blue quarters	Gas	137	7
Air	Grey	White/black quarters	Gas	137	1,5
Carbon dioxide	Grey	Grey	Liquid and vapour	50	2,6/1,6
Oxygen/helium	Black	White/brown quarters	Gas	137	4,6/2,4

*Note that all gas-containing cylinders are filled to 137 bar; the pressure in vapour-containing cylinders is the Saturated vapour pressure of the liquid at room temperature (15°C).

Al-Shaikh B and Stacey S (2006) *Essentials of Anaesthetic Equipment*, 3rd edition. Edinburgh: Churchill Livingstone.
BOC Medical. Medical gas cylinder data chart. Available at: www.bocmedical.co.uk.
Kevin K and Spoors C (2009) *Training in Anaesthesia*. New York: Oxford University Press.

24 Heat and moisture exchange (HME) humidifiers:

a **False** They can provide relative humidity of 60–70%.
b **False** Inspired gases are warmed to between 29°C and 34°C.
c **True** The greater the temperature difference between each side of the HME filter, the greater the potential for heat and moisture to be transferred during inspiration and expiration.
d **False** The increase in dead space could be up to 100 ml in adults.
e **False** HME filters have a pore size of 0.2 μm for this purpose.

Al-Shaikh B and Stacey S (2006) *Essentials of Anaesthetic Equipment*, 3rd edition. Edinburgh: Churchill Livingstone.

25 Concerning temperature:

a **True** Although the values are different, the intervals on the scale are equivalent.
b **True** The Kelvin is defined as 1/273.16 of the thermodynamic temperature of the triple point of water. Temperature in Kelvin is equal to the temperature in Celsius plus 273.15.
c **False** The triple point of water occurs at 0.01°C.
d **False** The triple point of water is the temperature at which ice, water, and water vapour are in equilibrium.
e **True** The temperature of a gas is a measure of the speed of movement of its molecules. The higher the temperature the more heat energy is transferred to the gas and the greater the movement of the molecules.

Davis P and Kenny G (2002) *Basic Physics and Measurement in Anaesthesia*, 5th edition. Boston, MA: Butterworth-Heinemann.

26 Regarding temperature measurement:

a **False** In the resistance wire thermometer a metal wire, often platinum, is used. It works on the principle that the electrical resistance of the wire increases as the temperature increases.

b **False** It is the thermocouple that utilizes the Seebeck effect.

c **True** The thermocouple uses two dissimilar metals, e.g. copper and constantan. Where they join a small voltage is produced This is the Seebeck effect. A second junction is used to complete the circuit. One junction (reference) is kept at a constant temperature and the other junction is used in the temperature probe.

d **False** Alcohol thermometers are used to measure very low temperatures as mercury freezes at –39°C.

e **False** The thermistor contains a bead of metal oxide. The resistance of the thermistor falls exponentially with an increase in temperature, in contrast to the resistance thermometer.

Al-Shaikh B and Stacey S (2006) *Essentials of Anaesthetic Equipment*, 3rd edition. Edinburgh: Churchill Livingstone.

27 The classic laryngeal mask airway (LMA™):

a **True** Not all of the disposable models currently available are made of silicone and consequently may not be as easy to introduce, and can be more abrasive than reusable models.

b **False** The manufacturer suggests a maximum of 40 uses. However damage by patients' teeth may mean that their effective lifespan is much less than this.

c **True** Laryngeal masks with non-metallic self sealing valves are now available for use in the MRI scanner.

d **False** Although LMAs have wide internal diameters, their range varies from 7 mm to 10, 10, and 11.5, mm for sizes 2, 3, 4, and 5, respectively.

e **True** This is in contrast to armoured endotracheal tubes, which are often reinforced with strands of nylon.

Al-Shaikh B and Stacey S (2006) *Essentials of Anaesthetic Equipment*, 3rd edition. Edinburgh: Churchill Livingstone.

28 The Clark electrode:

a **False** It can measure the oxygen tension in the blood sample.

b **True** A platinum cathode and a silver/silver chloride anode are placed in an electrolyte solution, e.g. potassium chloride. A voltage of 0.6 V is applied between the electrodes and the current flow is measured. The current is proportional to the amount of oxygen present. The blood sample is separated from the electrodes by a Teflon membrane to prevent protein deposits forming on the electrode.

c **False** It has a slower response time as the oxygen must diffuse across the membrane.

d **True** The Clark or polarographic oxygen analyser can measure the oxygen in gas, but its response time is slow and it gives only an average of the inspired and expired concentrations

e **False** It has a life expectancy of three years due to deterioration of the membrane. The membrane must be checked regularly to ensure its integrity and lack of protein deposits.

Al-Shaikh B and Stacey S (2006) *Essentials of Anaesthetic Equipment*, 3rd edition. Edinburgh: Churchill Livingstone.

29 Concerning cylinder valves:

a **False** They are made of brass and are sometimes chromium plated.
b **True** The content of the cylinder type is engraved on the cylinder neck.
c **False** The pin index position for oxygen is 2 and 5 and for nitrous oxide is 3 and 5. For air, the position is 1 and 5.
d **True** Otherwise there could be the risk of an explosion.
e **True** The Bodok seal is a compressible washer which must in good condition and placed properly to prevent leakage.

Al-Shaikh B and Stacey S (2006) *Essentials of Anaesthetic Equipment*, 3rd edition. Edinburgh: Churchill Livingstone.

30 Methods of non-invasive blood pressure monitoring include:

a **True** Simple palpation of the pulse during release of cuff pressure can give the systolic pressure.
b **True** The Riva–Rocci method uses the cuff and auscultation over the artery to detect the Korotkoff sounds.
c **True** It was the precursor of the automatic blood pressure monitors. Measurements can be made remotely from the patient without the need for auscultation of the arterial pulse. The Von Recklinghausen oscillotonometer is an example.
d **True** Unlike the oscillotonometer, electric oscillometric equipment uses a single cuff only. Oscillometers are automated blood pressure measuring devices, an example is the DINAMAP (device for indirect non-invasive automatic mean arterial pressure). The frequency of measurements can be set and a visual reading is displayed.
e **False** This is a method of measuring cardiac output (impedance plethysmography) and is also used in respiratory function tests (body plethysmography). It is not routinely used for the measurement of blood pressure.

Aitkenhead A and Smith G (2008) *Textbook of Anaesthesia*, 5th edition. Edinburgh: Churchill Livingstone.
Al-Shaikh B and Stacey S (2006) *Essentials of Anaesthetic Equipment*, 3rd edition. Edinburgh: Churchill Livingstone.

chapter 3

PHYSIOLOGY

QUESTIONS

1 Stimulation of alpha adrenergic receptors causes:

a Tachycardia
b Vasodilation
c Uterine relaxation
d Increased intestinal tone
e Relaxation of the bladder sphincter

2 Regarding lung function tests:

a Spirometry can be used to accurately predict pulmonary complications
b Normal ratio between forced expiratory volume in one second and forced vital capacity (FEV_1:FVC ratio) is approximately 80%
c Peak flow is useful in detecting a restrictive lung disorder
d Normal peak flow in an adult male would be 5 l/kg body weight
e An FEV_1 of <1 litre indicates poor postoperative lung function necessitating respiratory support

3 Features of hypermagnesaemia include:

a Blood levels of >2.5 mmol/l
b Tachycardia
c Hypertension
d Respiratory depression
e Impaired clotting

4 Hyponatraemia:

a Is present when plasma sodium levels are <120 mmol/l
b May be caused by excessive diuretic use
c May be secondary to malignancy
d May be secondary to hyperglycaemia
e May cause cerebral oedema

5 Regarding renal function:

a Creatinine is a product of skeletal muscle metabolism
b Creatinine clearance reflects glomerular filtration rate (GFR)
c A small change in serum creatinine implies a large change in GFR
d GFR falls by 1% per annum after 30 years of age
e Uraemia affects platelet function and bleeding time may be prolonged

6 Insulin:

a Is secreted by the alpha cells in the pancreas
b Inhibits lipolysis, proteolysis, and glycogenolysis
c Dosage may have to be increased if the glycosylated haemoglobin ($HbA1_c$) is between 4% and 5%
d Is necessary even while fasting to maintain glucose homeostasis by counteracting stress hormones such as adrenaline (epinephrine)
e May be adsorbed onto infusion bags

7 In hypothyroidism:

a Thyroid-stimulating hormone (TSH) secretion is abnormally high
b T_4 levels are low
c Antithyroid antibodies may be present
d Low blood pressure is a feature
e Tachycardia is a feature

8 Metabolic functions of the lung include:

a Surfactant production
b Conversion of angiotensin I to angiotensin II
c Inactivation of bradykinin
d Inactivation of 5-hydroxytryptamine
e Inactivation of prostaglandins

9 Regarding red blood cells:

a The total number is 2.5×10^{12}
b They are 10–12 μm in diameter
c Packed cell volume (PCV) is 0.37–0.47 in women
d Most are released as reticulocytes initially
e The average lifespan is 90 days

10 Regarding the oxyhaemoglobin dissociation curve:

a P50 is when haemoglobin is fully saturated at a PaO_2 of 50 kPa
b P50 is the PaO_2 at which haemoglobin is 50% saturated
c A shift either to the right or left occurs from a fixed PaO_2 of 6kPa
d A fall in 2,3-DPG shifts the curve to the right
e The dissociation curve of fetal haemoglobin is to the right of the adult haemoglobin curve

11 In a lower motor neuron lesion:

a Denervation of muscles below the level of lesion occurs
b Tendon reflexes are weak or absent
c Babinski's reflex is present
d Proprioception, vibration, and fine touch are preserved on the side of lesion
e Is a contraindication to the use of depolarizing relaxants

12 In the autonomic nervous system:

- a Sympathetic preganglionic fibres secrete noradrenaline (norepinephrine)
- b Sympathetic stimulation causes pupillary constriction
- c Acetylcholine receptors in both sympathetic and parasympathetic ganglia are nicotinic
- d Vagal nerve stimulation decreases gastric motility
- e The adrenal medulla secretes adrenaline (epinephrine) in response to stimulation of the postganglionic fibres in the splanchnic nerves

13 In hypercalcaemia:

- a Serum calcium is greater than 2.5 mmol/l
- b Arrhythmias occur
- c Thiazide diuretics are the recommended treatment
- d Calcitonin increases calcium excretion
- e Muscle fasciculations may be present

14 Concerning thyroid gland function:

- a Thyroxine is derived from tyrosine
- b Iodine attached to position 3 and 5 on tyrosine gives mono and diiodothyronine, respectively
- c Interaction between mono- and diiodothyronine gives triiodothyronine (T_3) and thyroxine (T_4)
- d Thyroxine decreases the sensitivity of beta adrenergic receptors
- e Thyroxine antagonizes the effects of insulin

15 Regarding platelets:

- a A count of 150×10^9/l is normal
- b They are 6–8 μm in diameter
- c They secrete adenosine diphosphate (ADP) and 5-hydroxytryptamine (5HT) and form a plug at the site of injury
- d They may predispose to spontaneous bleeding at levels of $60–70 \times 10^9$/l
- e Dysfunction is the cause of bleeding in von Willebrand's disease

16 The following are involved in the metabolism of adrenaline (epinephrine):

- a Catechol-*O*-methyl transferase (COMT)
- b Monoamine oxidase (MAO)
- c 5-hydroxytryptamine
- d Hydroxybutyric acid
- e Dihydroxyphenylalanine

17 The diffusing capacity of the lungs:

- a Is also described as the transfer factor
- b Can be measured by the single breath method using 0.3% carbon monoxide and 10% helium
- c It is decreased in lung fibrosis
- d Is unaffected by emphysema
- e Has a normal value of 12–15 ml/min/mmHg

18 Ions with a greater intracellular concentration compared with extracellular concentration include:

a Sodium
b Chloride
c Magnesium
d Potassium
e Bicarbonate

19 Hypokalaemia:

a May produce intestinal ileus
b May be accompanied by a compensatory increase in aldosterone secretion
c May produce muscle rigidity
d Produces T wave inversion and prolonged P-R interval on the electrocardiogram (ECG)
e Is associated with a metabolic alkalosis

20 In the lungs:

a Blood flow is greatest at the base in the erect position
b Alveolar PO_2 is greatest at the apex of the lungs
c Compliance is greater in the dependent lung in the lateral position in the awake patient.
d Ventilation and perfusion are matched in the mid zone
e Blood from the non-ventilated parts of the lung is diverted to the ventilated areas in hypoxic pulmonary vasoconstriction

21 In the postoperative stress response:

a Growth hormone levels increase
b Corticosteroid production decreases
c Glucagon levels are elevated
d Insulin resistance occurs
e ADH levels increase

22 The following antagonize the action of insulin:

a Growth hormone
b Adrenaline (epinephrine)
c Oestrogens
d Biguanides
e Sulphonylureas

23 Bowel peristalsis is increased by:

a Anticholinesterases
b Sympathetic blockade
c Atropine
d Adrenaline (epinephrine)
e Hyoscine

24 Pituitary hormones include:

a TSH
b ACTH
c Prolactin
d Dopamine
e Somatostatin

25 The hypothalamus:

a Controls body temperature
b Contains the vasomotor centre situated in the anterior hypothalamus
c Secretes melanocyte stimulating hormone (MSH)
d Controls thirst
e Controls hunger

26 The kidneys:

a Produce erythropoietin
b Secrete renin
c Produce 1,25 dihydroxycholecalciferol
d Synthesize prostaglandins
e Normally produce urine with a pH of between 7.7 and 8

27 Concerning white blood cells:

a A normal count is 2–4 × 10^9/l
b Neutrophils form around 40–75% of total white cells
c Lymphocytes make up approximately a third of the total white cells
d Eosinophils contribute less than 8% of the total white cells
e Monocytes constitute less than 1% of the total white cells

28 Hypothermia:

a Exists when a patient has a core temperature of 35°C
b Can increase surgical bleeding
c Increases the peripheral vascular resistance
d Predisposes to arrhythmias at temperatures below 32°C
e Can protect the brain for longer periods in low cardiac output states

29 Concerning renal function:

a Urine concentration of urea is greater than plasma urea
b Normal plasma urea:creatinine ratio is 10:1
c Renal clearance is defined as the volume of plasma completely cleared of a substance in one minute
d Inulin clearance is used for measuring GFR
e The urine normally contains no glucose

30 Dopamine:

a Is a precursor of L–dopa
b Is a neurotransmitter
c Deficiency results in the bradykinesia and rigidity seen in Parkinsonism
d Improves renal blood flow in low doses
e Is also known as prolactin inhibiting factor (PIF)

chapter 3 PHYSIOLOGY

ANSWERS

1 Stimulation of alpha adrenergic receptors causes:

a **False** There is increased vasoconstriction but no direct effect on the heart rate.

b **False** Stimulation of the alpha 1 receptors causes contraction of vascular smooth muscle and therefore vasoconstriction.

c **False** Beta stimulation produces uterine relaxation in the gravid uterus, whereas alpha stimulation has a variable effect in the non-gravid uterus and may produce premature contractions in the gravid uterus.

d **False** There is an overall decrease in intestinal tone and motility although the sphincters may be contracted.

e **False** Alpha receptor stimulation increases the tone of the urethral sphincter. Ephedrine, which is a weak alpha and beta agonist has been responsible for producing urinary retention in older male patients taking over-the-counter cough mixtures containing ephedrine.

Barrett K, Barman S, Boitano S, and Brooks HL (2009) *Ganong's Review of Medical Physiology*, 23rd edition. USA: McGraw-Hill.

2 Regarding lung function tests:

a **False** Lung function tests are only a guide to the patient's ability to cope postoperatively, but cannot accurately predict the possible complications. There is a training effect and there may be considerable intra-subject variation, so the results may not accurately reflect their true lung function.

b **True** A ratio of FEV_1:FVC of approximately 80% is normal. The ratio is reduced in obstructive lung disorders. In restrictive lung disorders the FEV_1 may be reduced, but as the FVC is also reduced, the ratio of FEV_1 to FVC may be normal, or even increased. Middle-aged patients will often have an FEV_1:FVC ratio of around 70–75% and at age 70 it could be as low as 65%. These variations with age have to be borne in mind before interpreting the results.

c **False** When the lung is either compressed from the outside by tumour, pneumothorax, or pleural effusion, all the lung function tests are reduced, but the ratios would still remain the same. Since the peak flow meter records the maximum expiratory flow per minute it is a better guide to an obstructive disorder.

d **False** A rough approximation is between 7 l/kg and 10 l/kg body weight.

e **True** At this level coughing and clearance of secretions would be poor especially in the postoperative period. A patient like this would need managing postoperatively in a high-dependency nursing environment.

Allman K and Wilson I (2006) *Oxford Handbook of Anaesthesia*, 2nd edition. New York: Oxford University Press

3 Features of hypermagnesaemia include:

a **True** Normal levels for magnesium are 0.7–1 mmol/l. Hypermagnesaemia is a level greater than 2.5 mmol/l. There may be limited value in measuring serum levels, however, as most magnesium is intracellular.

b **False** The normal picture is a prolonged P-R interval, widened QRS complexes. Bradycardia and cardiac arrest may occur at levels greater than 15 mmol/l.

c **False** Vasodilation and hypotension are common features.

d **True** Along with central nervous system (CNS) symptoms of sedation, coma and muscle weakness, respiratory depression is common.

e **True** Clotting may be affected because of the imbalance between magnesium and calcium ions.

Allman K, McIndoe A, and Wilson I (2009) *Emergencies in Anaesthesia*. 2nd edition. New York: Oxford University Press.

4 Hyponatraemia:

a **True** At this level it is classified as severe hyponatraemia. Normal levels are 135–145 mmol/l. A level of 125–134 mmol/l is considered mild and 120–124 mmol/l is moderate hyponatraemia.

b **True** Excessive use of diuretics in the first instance will produce volume depletion, which in turn stimulates antidiuretic hormone (ADH) secretion and water retention, and consequently hyponatraemia.

c **True** Certain tumours, e.g. lung (small cell carcinoma), may be responsible for a syndrome of inappropriate antidiuretic hormone (SIADH) release and water retention with hyponatraemia.

d **True** Hyperglycaemia reduces serum sodium by 1.5 mmol/l for every 3.5 mmol/l rise in plasma glucose. The hyponatraemia is caused by a redistribution of sodium and water. Water shifts from the intracellular to the extracellular compartment causing an apparent hyponatraemia but the total body water and sodium concentrations remain the same. To calculate the corrected plasma sodium concentration the formula is: (sodium) + (glucose/4).

e **True** A severe state of hyponatraemia may cause an osmotic shift of water from the plasma to the brain cells, causing cerebral oedema.

Allman K, McIndoe A, and Wilson I (2009) *Emergencies in Anaesthesia*, 2nd edition. New York: Oxford University Press.
Yentis S, Hirsh N, and Smith G (2003) *Anaesthesia and Intensive Care A to Z*, 3rd edition. London: Butterworth-Heinemann.

5 Regarding renal function:

a **True** Creatinine is formed mainly in skeletal muscle from phosphorylcreatine (from adenosine triphosphate (ATP) and creatine).

b **True** Since there is very little renal tubular secretion of creatinine, its renal clearance reflects the GFR. Creatinine production also remains fairly constant, therefore, plasma levels are an accurate reflection of renal function. Serial values are of most use.

c **True** Plasma creatinine shows a rectangular hyperbolic relationship with creatinine clearance, i.e. GFR must fall by 50% before serum creatinine begins to rise. Therefore a small change in serum creatinine must imply a large change in GFR.

d **True** It has been shown that GFR falls progressively with age. Normal GFR is 90–130 ml/min. There is renal failure when the GFR is <15 ml/min.

e **True** Although the platelet count may be normal, the platelet function may be abnormal as a result of renal impairment and the bleeding time may be prolonged. This may also be seen on thromboelastography (TEG) studies of coagulation.

Allman K and Wilson I (2006) *Oxford Handbook of Anaesthesia*, 2nd edition. New York: Oxford University Press.

6 Insulin:

a **False** It is secreted by the beta cells of the islets of Langerhans in the pancreas.

b **True** Insulin increases glucose uptake, glycogen synthesis, fat synthesis, protein synthesis, and potassium uptake. Insulin decreases glycogen breakdown, gluconeogenesis, lipolysis, proteolysis, and hepatic ketone body formation. The overall effect is a decrease in blood glucose and increased utilization of glucose.

c **False** Glucose attaches to haemoglobin, allowing measurement of $HbA1_c$ or glycosylated haemoglobin which represents the average blood glucose levels over the previous 120 days, the lifespan of the red blood cell. The figure in per cent roughly equates to the average blood glucose in mmol/l. Normal levels of glycated haemoglobin in a non-diabetic person are 3.5–5.5%. A level of around 6.5% is good in diabetes. Levels above 7% indicate that control could be optimized and above 9% suggests inadequate control.

d **True** All other hormones including adrenaline (epinephrine) tend to stimulate glucose release and therefore insulin is required to counteract their effects. This is why a basal level of insulin is required even in the fasting state to prevent ketone formation.

e **True** This is due to the physical incompatibility exhibited by the insulin towards the plasticizers of the infusion bag and the administration set. Manufacturers are now making infusion bags without the need for plasticizers. Insulin is used in infusion bags in the GKI (glucose, potassium, and insulin) regimens without problems. A syringe driver system may be used for an insulin sliding scale regimen where tighter control of blood glucose is required.

Allman K and Wilson I (2006) *Oxford Handbook of Anaesthesia*, 2nd edition. New York: Oxford University Press.

7 In hypothyroidism:

a **True** It signifies reduced thyroid function, and therefore the TSH levels are raised.

b **True** T_4 is thyroxine and would be low. Levels of T_3 (triiodothyronine) are also low.

c **True** One of the causes of the disease is an autoimmune destruction of the thyroid gland and antibodies may be seen in the blood. Other causes are following hyperthyroidism treatment and side effects of amiodarone and lithium. Hypothyroidism may be secondary to pituitary disease, although this is rare.

d **True** Low circulating volume and low blood pressure are the usual features.

e **False** Low cardiac output, bradycardia, hypotension, and ischaemic heart disease are common findings.

Allman K and Wilson I (2006) *Oxford Handbook of Anaesthesia*, 2nd edition. New York: Oxford University Press.

Yentis S, Hirsh N, and Smith G (2003) *Anaesthesia and Intensive Care A to Z*, 3rd edition. London: Butterworth-Heinemann.

8 Metabolic functions of the lung include:

a **True** Surfactant is a fluid layer, secreted by the type II pneumocytes of the alveoli, lining the alveoli. The surfactant reduces the pressure required to hold the alveoli open, and minimizes the tendency of the small alveoli to collapse.

b **True** The conversion of angiotensin I to angiotensin II occurs mostly in the lungs, mediated by angiotensin converting enzyme (ACE).

c **True** Bradykinin is also broken down by angiotensin-converting enzyme (ACE) in the lungs. ACE inhibitor use may not be tolerated due to a build-up of bradykinin producing a chronic dry cough.

d **True** The lung receives all of the cardiac output and as such is well placed to metabolize or deactivate circulating compounds. In addition to angiotensin and bradykinin, the lungs also metabolize 5-hydroxytryptamine and take up amide local anaesthetics.

e **True** Prostaglandins have only a short half-life and are metabolized in the pulmonary, hepatic, and renal circulations along with local destruction.

Barrett K, Barman S, Boitano S, and Brooks HL (2009) *Ganong's Review of Medical Physiology*, 23rd edition. USA: McGraw-Hill.

Yentis S, Hirsh N, and Smith G (2003) *Anaesthesia and Intensive Care A to Z*, 3rd edition. London: Butterworth-Heinemann.

9 Regarding red blood cells:

a **False** The normal red blood cell count is 4.5–6.5 × 10^{12} in men and 3.9–5.6 × 10^{12} in women.

b **False** They are 2 μm thick and 8 μm in diameter.

c **True** The PCV or haematocrit is the total red cell volume as a fraction of the total blood volume and is 0.4–0.54 in men and 0.37–0.47 in women.

d **True** The transition is from erythroblast to reticulocyte and then to erythrocyte. The whole process takes seven days and is stimulated by erythropoietin. The change from reticulocyte to erythrocyte takes less than a day. Sites of erythropoiesis in an adult include the iliac crests, long bones, vertebrae, sternum, and ribs.

e **False** The average lifespan of an erythrocyte is approximately 120 days.

Allman K and Wilson I (2006) *Oxford Handbook of Anaesthesia*, 2nd edition. New York: Oxford University Press.

Pocock G and Richards C (2004) *Human Physiology: The basis of medicine*, 3rd edition. Oxford: Oxford University Press.

10 Regarding the oxyhaemoglobin dissociation curve:

a **False** P50 is the point on the oxyhaemoglobin dissociation curve when haemoglobin is 50% saturated, normally at a PO_2 of 3.5 kPa.

b **True** The P50 can be used as a reference point on the curve.

c **False** The oxyhaemoglobin dissociation curve can be described as shifting left or right from the P50 reference point where PO_2 is 3.5 kPa.

d **False** An increase in 2,3-DPG shifts the curve to the right (P50 >3.5 kPa). Other factors causing a right shift include acidosis, increase in temperature, and increase in carbon dioxide. Saturation is lower for a given PO_2 and oxygen is unloaded to the tissues more readily. The opposite situations cause a leftward shift and favour haemoglobin binding of oxygen.

e **False** The dissociation curve is further to the left in the fetus as well as in methaemoglobinaemia and carbon monoxide poisoning.

Barrett K, Barman S, Boitano S, and Brooks HL (2009) *Ganong's Review of Medical Physiology*, 23rd edition. USA: McGraw-Hill.

Cross M and Plunkett E (2008) *Physics, Pharmacology and Physiology for Anaesthetists*. Cambridge: Cambridge University Press.

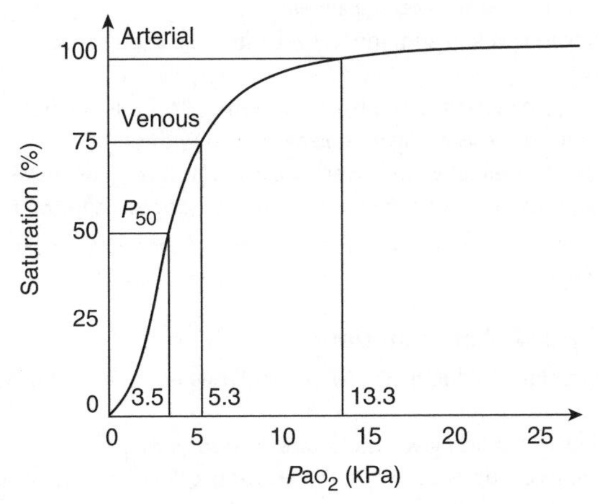

Figure 3.4 Oxyhaemoglobin dissociation curve.
Reproduced with kind permission from Cross M and Plunkett E (2008) *Physics, Pharmacology and Physiology for Anaesthetists*. Cambridge: Cambridge University Press.

11 In a lower motor neurone lesion:

a **True** Muscle tone is lost in the initial period and may be followed later by spasticity.

b **True** This is particularly true in the acute phase.

c **False** Babinski's reflex is seen in an upper motor neurone lesion and involves dorsiflexion and fanning of the toes.

d **False** Proprioception, vibration, and fine touch sensations are lost on the side of lesion.

e **True** Where a lower motor neurone lesion has occurred there can be denervation hypersensitivity as acetylcholine receptors become distributed throughout the entire muscle, which can lead to a rise in serum potassium of several millimoles per litre when fasciculation occurs.

Barrett K, Barman S, Boitano S, and Brooks HL (2009) *Ganong's Review of Medical Physiology*, 23rd edition. USA: McGraw-Hill.

Yentis S, Hirsh N, and Smith G (2003) *Anaesthesia and Intensive Care A to Z*, 3rd edition. London: Butterworth-Heinemann.

12 In the autonomic nervous system:

a **False** The preganglionic fibres secrete acetylcholine in both the sympathetic and parasympathetic systems.
b **False** Constriction of the pupil is governed by the parasympathetic nervous system, via the oculomotor nerve and the ciliary ganglion and short ciliary nerves.
c **True** Both ganglia are nicotinic in function.
d **False** Vagal stimulation increases gastric secretion and motility. This was the basis for vagotomy in the treatment of peptic ulcer disease before the introduction of proton pump inhibitors.
e **False** The adrenaline (epinephrine) secretion is in response to preganglionic fibres in the splanchnic nerves.

Barrett K, Barman S, Boitano S, and Brooks HL (2009) *Ganong's Review of Medical Physiology*, 23rd edition. USA: McGraw-Hill.

13 In hypercalcaemia:

a **True** Normal serum calcium is 2.2–2.5 mmol/l. Levels greater than 2.5 mmol/l constitute mild hypercalcaemia. Moderate hypercalcaemia is 3.0–3.4 mmol/l and greater than 3.4 mmol/l is severe hypercalcaemia.
b **True** Prolonged P-R and shortened Q-T intervals and bradycardia may be seen as well as dysrhythmias.
c **False** They may exacerbate the hypercalcaemia. Loop diuretics, e.g. furosemide, may be used to promote diuresis along with rehydration with saline.
d **True** Calcitonin is effective in lowering calcium levels by decreasing bone resorption.
e **True** Muscle fasciculations may be particularly noticeable in the tongue.

Allman K, McIndoe A, and Wilson I (2009) *Emergencies in Anaesthesia*, 2nd edition. New York: Oxford University Press.

14 Concerning thyroid gland function:

a **True** The tyrosine residue from thyroglobulin when iodinated produces mono-iodotyrosine.
b **False** Further iodination gives mono and diiodotyrosine.
c **True** Coupling reactions between the above produces the thyronines.
d **False** Thyroxine acts to increase tissue metabolism and growth, it also increases the number of beta adrenergic receptors and their sensitivity to circulating catecholamines.
e **False** Thyroxine potentiates the effects of insulin, enhances the intestinal absorption of glucose, and increases the rate of glucose uptake by muscle and adipose tissue.

Barrett K, Barman S, Boitano S, and Brooks HL (2009) *Ganong's Review of Medical Physiology*, 23rd edition. USA: McGraw-Hill.

15 Platelets:

a **True** The normal platelet count is 150–400 × 10^9/l. Below 150 is defined as thrombocytopenia.

b **False** They are 2–4 μm in diameter.

c **True** Within seconds of a vascular injury, platelets start to aggregate and adhere to the site of damage. They release a number of substances from their cytoplasmic granules including ADP and 5HT, and in addition synthesize and release arachidonic acid and thromboxane A_2. Collectively, they change the surface characteristics of the platelets causing them to adhere to the vessel wall and to each other.

d **False** Spontaneous bleeding is uncommon until the count falls below 10–20 × 10^9/l. When they reach this level haemorrhage may occur from oral and other mucous membranes, the gastrointestinal tract, or an intracerebral event may occur.

e **True** von Willebrand's disease is the commonest inherited coagulation disorder. There are three subtypes of the disease. The majority of cases are autosomal dominant, however, there is an autosomal recessive form. It is caused by abnormal von Willebrand's factor, which usually aids platelet adhesion and factor VIII carriage. The effects are a reduction in factor VIII, abnormality of platelet adhesion, and an abnormal epithelium, leading to an increased tendency to bleed.

Allman K and Wilson I (2006) *Oxford Handbook of Anaesthesia*, 2nd edition. New York: Oxford University Press.

Barrett K, Barman S, Boitano S, and Brooks HL (2009) *Ganong's Review of Medical Physiology*, 23rd edition. USA: McGraw-Hill.

16 The following are involved in the metabolism of adrenaline (epinephrine):

a **True** COMT is the enzyme that catalyses the conversion of adrenaline (epinephrine) to metanephrine, which is then converted to 4-hydroxy 3-methoxy mandelic acid (HMMA) and vanillylmandelic acid (VMA), which is excreted in the urine. VMA estimation in the urine has been used as a test for the diagnosis of phaeochromocytoma.

b **True** MAO is the enzyme involved in catalysing the metabolism of catecholamines at nerve endings.

c **False** 5-HT is serotonin and is not involved in the biodegradation of adrenaline (epinephrine).

d **False** Acetoacetic acid and hydroxybutyric acid are known as ketone bodies, the accumulation of which is responsible for the acidosis seen in uncontrolled diabetes.

e **False** Dihydroxyphenylalanine (DOPA) is a precursor which is broken down by the action of DOPA decarboxylase to produce dopamine, which is then converted to either noradrenaline (norepinephrine) or adrenaline (epinephrine).

Barrett K, Barman S, Boitano S, and Brooks HL (2009) *Ganong's Review of Medical Physiology*, 23rd edition. USA: McGraw-Hill.

17 The diffusing capacity of the lungs:

a **True** Both terms define the functional integrity of the alveoli.

b **True** This is one of the ways of measuring the transfer of gases. Carbon monoxide is frequently used as its uptake is diffusion limited. A single inspiration of carbon monoxide is made and the rate of decrease in carbon monoxide from the alveolar gas during a 10–20 second breath hold is measured. Helium is added to the inspired mixture so that the lung volume can be estimated by helium dilution. An infrared analyser is then used to calculate the difference between the inspired and expired carbon monoxide concentrations.

Another method is continuous breathing of carbon monoxide 0.3% for up to one minute. The rate of uptake of carbon monoxide is measured when the steady state is reached.

c **True** When the lung parenchyma is diseased or destroyed the gas exchange will be severely affected. Both obstructive and restrictive lung disorders cause a reduction in diffusing capacity.

d **False** Emphysema is a chronic condition in which there is progressive destruction and dilatation of the alveoli, and diffusing capacity is reduced.

e **False** The normal value is 17–25 ml/min/mmHg. Diffusing capacity increases during exercise as a result of recruitment and distension of pulmonary capillaries.

Allman K and Wilson I (2006) *Oxford Handbook of Anaesthesia*, 2nd edition. New York: Oxford University Press.

West J (2004) *Respiratory Physiology*, 7th edition. Philadelphia: Lippincott Williams and Wilkins.

18 Ions with a greater intracellular concentration compared with extracellular concentration include:

a **False** Remember for example that sodium ions are outside the nerve membrane and enter the nerve only in response to a stimulus when the sodium channels open. The total extracellular sodium is 91%, and the intracellular portion is 9%.

b **False** The majority of chloride is extracellular. The normal plasma chloride concentration is 95–105 mmol/l. Intracellular chloride is 3 mmol/l and the extracellular concentration is 117 mmol/l.

c **True** It is the second most abundant intracellular cation. 99% of magnesium is intracellular and 1% is extracellular. Normal plasma levels are 0.75–1.05 mmol/l.

d **True** Potassium is the main intracellular cation. 90% of the potassium is intracellular, 7.5% is found in bone and connective tissue, and only 2.5% is in the interstitial fluid. Intracellular levels are 135–150 mmol/l, whereas in the plasma the concentration is 3.5–5.0 mmol/l.

e **False** Most of the bicarbonate is extracellular and carried in the plasma at a normal concentration of 24–33 mmol/l and is formed from the dissociation of carbonic acid.

Barrett K, Barman S, Boitano S, and Brooks HL (2009) *Ganong's Review of Medical Physiology*, 23rd edition. USA: McGraw-Hill.

Pinnock C, Lin T, and Smith T (2002) *Fundamentals of Anaesthesia*, 2nd edition. New York: Cambridge University Press.

19 Hypokalaemia:

a **True** Intestinal atony is seen in hypokalaemia, which should be excluded before embarking on any surgical intervention.

b **False** There is decreased aldosterone release to enable renal preservation of potassium. The is an excess of aldosterone and hypokalaemia in hyperaldosteronism (Conn's syndrome).

c **False** There is muscle weakness and increased sensitivity to neuromuscular blocking drugs.

d **True** The ECG features include ST depression, increase in P-R and Q-T intervals, and T wave inversion. There may be a U wave present. Cardiac arrest may occur.

e **True** Hypokalaemia is associated with metabolic alkalosis. For each 0.1 increase in pH the potassium decreases by 0.6 mmol/l.

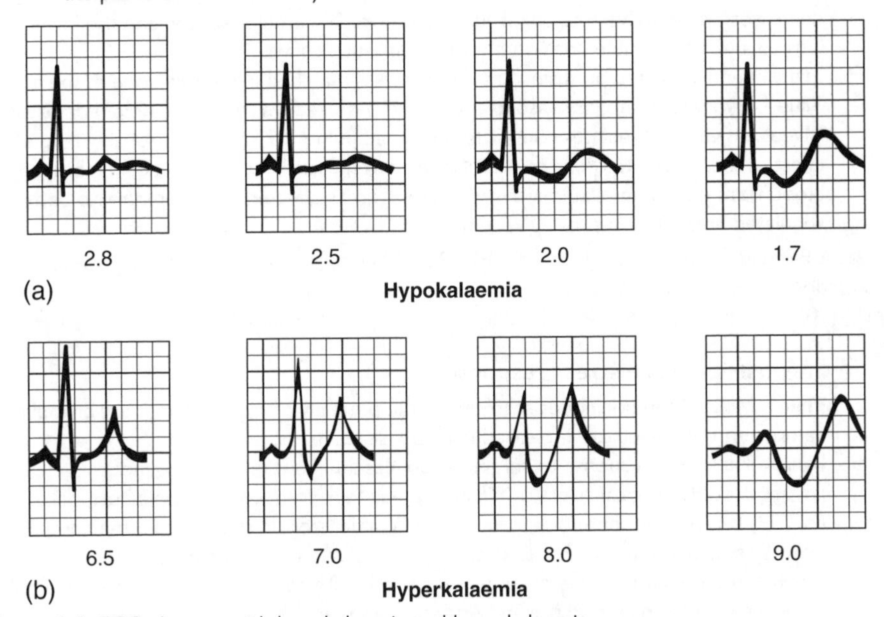

Figure 3.5 ECG changes with hypokalaemia and hyperkalaemia.
Reproduced with kind permission from Kevin K and Spoors C (2009) *Training in Anaesthesia*. New York: Oxford University Press.

Allman K and Wilson I (2006) *Oxford Handbook of Anaesthesia*, 2nd edition. New York: Oxford University Press.

20 In the lungs:

a **True** It is least at the apex in the erect position and greatest in the base. The decrease in blood flow from the base to the apex of the lungs is almost linear in the upright position. The difference is due to varying hydrostatic pressure within the pulmonary vessels.

b **True** As the apex has better ventilation in comparison with blood flow, the partial pressure of oxygen is high. There is a ventilation/perfusion (V/Q) mismatch where ventilation is greater than perfusion.

c **True** When an awake patient changes from the supine to the lateral decubitus position, the lower lung maintains good ventilation as it moves to a more favourable position on the compliance curve. The upper lung is in a less favourable position on the curve. However, when the patient is anaesthetized, the functional residual capacity decreases, which moves the upper lung to a more favourable position and the lower lung to a less favourable position on the compliance curve.

d **True** Ventilation and perfusion are more or less matched in the mid-zone of the lungs.

e **True** Hypoxic pulmonary vasoconstriction is a protective reflex in pulmonary disease. Alveolar hypoxia stimulates constriction of small pulmonary arteries probably by the effect of local mediators on the vascular smooth muscle. The overall effect is to direct blood from poorly ventilated areas of lung, e.g. areas affected by pneumonia, to better ventilated areas thus improving V/Q mismatch overall.

Barrett K, Barman S, Boitano S, and Brooks HL (2009) *Ganong's Review of Medical Physiology*, 23rd edition. USA: McGraw-Hill.
West J (2004) *Respiratory Physiology*, 7th edition. Philadelphia: Lippincott Williams and Wilkins.

21 In the postoperative stress response:

a **True** Most of the hormones secreted by the pituitary or hypothalamus are anabolic in nature and their levels are increased in response to stress.

b **False** The stress response to surgery produces an elevation in endogenous corticosteroids. Surgical stress or trauma stimulates adrenocorticotropic hormone (ACTH) release and therefore an increase in corticosteroid release from the adrenals. Plasma cortisol levels rise. For this reason it is important to remember steroid supplementation at the time of surgery for those with adrenal insufficiency, for example following long-term steroid use and Addison's disease.

c **True** Glucagon levels increase leading to increased plasma glucose levels.

d **True** During surgery and the perioperative period there is insufficient insulin release to match the stress response's tendency towards hyperglycaemia. There is also impaired insulin release from the beta cells and the tissue response to insulin is decreased, leading to a state of insulin resistance.

e **True** The surgical stress response stimulates the release of ADH as a protective measure leading to retention of water. The renin–angiotensin system is also activated, leading to increased conservation of sodium and increased loss of potassium in the urine. All of these effects aim to restore volume.

Desborough JP (2000) The stress response to trauma and surgery. *Br J Anaesth* **85**:109–17.
Barrett K, Barman S, Boitano S, and Brooks HL (2009) *Ganong's Review of Medical Physiology*, 23rd edition. USA: McGraw-Hill.

22 The following antagonize the action of insulin:

a **True** Growth hormone is an insulin antagonist, it inhibits gluconeogenesis. Its release is increased in hypoglycaemic states and it is inhibited by hyperglycaemia.

b **True** Adrenaline (epinephrine) stimulates alpha 1 receptors leading to glycogenolysis. It also stimulates lipolysis and gluconeogenesis. Adrenaline also decreases secretion of insulin and glucagon from the pancreas. The overall effect is to increase the blood sugar.

c **True** Oestrogens act as insulin antagonists. Other insulin antagonists include cortisol, glucagon, and T_4.

d **False** Biguanides, e.g. metformin are oral hypoglycaemic agents. They increase the peripheral sensitivity of the tissues to insulin. They act synergistically with endogenous insulin.

e **False** Sulphonylureas are also oral hypoglycaemics, for example glibenclamide, gliclazide, and glipizide. Their mode of action is to stimulate endogenous release of insulin by displacing insulin from the beta cells in the pancreas.

Barrett K, Barman S, Boitano S, and Brooks HL (2009) *Ganong's Review of Medical Physiology*, 23rd edition. USA: McGraw-Hill.
Peck T, Hill S, and Williams M (2004) *Pharmacology for Anaesthesia and Intensive Care*, 2nd edition. Cambridge: Cambridge University Press.

23 Bowel peristalsis is increased by:

a **True** Elevated levels of acetylcholine increase peristalsis. It is for this reason that surgeons have been opposed to the use of neostigmine in the reversal of neuromuscular blockade, as increased peristalsis in the bowel can threaten the integrity of a bowel anastomosis.

b **True** There is relative over-activity of the parasympathetic system, causing increase in tone and peristalsis in the intestines.

c **False** Antimuscarinic agents cause relaxation of the gut, and they are employed for this purpose during investigations where decreased gut motility and relaxation of sphincters is desirable, for example during endoscopic examinations. They are sometimes used when anastomoses are being fashioned during bowel surgery.

d **False** Adrenaline (epinephrine) causes an overall decrease in intestinal motility.

e **False** It is an antimuscarinic drug. Hyoscine butylbromide (Buscopan) is used in the treatment of intestinal colic as an antispasmodic.

Barrett K, Barman S, Boitano S, and Brooks HL (2009) *Ganong's Review of Medical Physiology*, 23rd edition. USA: McGraw-Hill.

24 Pituitary hormones include:

a **True** TSH controls thyroxine formation on a negative feedback system.

b **True** ACTH is released by the pituitary. To distinguish between primary adrenocortical failure and failure of the pituitary, a Synacthen test is performed.

c **True** Prolactin is responsible for promoting growth and maturation of the mammary glands during pregnancy and for maintenance of lactation post partum.

d **False** Dopamine is secreted by the hypothalamus.

e **False** Somatostatin, also known as growth hormone inhibiting hormone, is secreted by the hypothalamus.

Barrett K, Barman S, Boitano S, and Brooks HL (2009) *Ganong's Review of Medical Physiology*, 23rd edition. USA: McGraw-Hill.

25 The hypothalamus:

a **True** The preoptic area of the hypothalamus contains neurones whose rate of discharge increases markedly in response to a rise in core temperature while others respond to a fall in core temperature by reducing their rates of discharge. The afferent input comes from the peripheral (skin) and central (core) thermoreceptors.

b **False** The vasomotor centre is situated in the ventrolateral medulla oblongata near the floor of the fourth ventricle.

c **False** MSH is secreted by the pituitary. It is thought to be responsible for the synthesis of melanin pigment.

d **True** The osmoreceptors located in the anterior hypothalamus regulate the amount of ADH secreted by the posterior pituitary, increasing ADH release in response to dehydration and decreasing ADH during a water load.

e **True** The lateral hypothalamus contains a region known as the feeding centre. The satiety centre is located in the ventromedial hypothalamus. These work in conjunction with each other to control food intake.

Barrett K, Barman S, Boitano S, and Brooks HL (2009) *Ganong's Review of Medical Physiology*, 23rd edition. USA: McGraw-Hill.

26 The kidneys:

a **True** Erythropoietin is an important stimulator of erythropoiesis. Levels of erythropoietin are decreased in chronic renal failure and the patient may require subcutaneous injections of recombinant erythropoietin. Conversely renal tumours may produce excess erythropoietin leading to polycythaemia.

b **True** Renin is a hormone made and secreted by the juxtaglomerular apparatus of the renal tubule. It has a key role in blood pressure and fluid balance homeostasis. Secretion is stimulated by hypovolaemia and increases angiotensin I production from angiotensinogen.

c **True** It is also called calcitriol and is synthesized from vitamin D, and stimulates the absorption of calcium from the gut and calcification of the bones.

d **True** The kidneys produce prostaglandins from arachidonic acid in the renal cortex, the medullary interstitium, and collecting duct. The prostaglandins produced by the kidney are PGE_2, $PGF_{2\alpha}$, PGD_2 and thromboxane A_2. The overall effect of the prostaglandins is to increase renal vasodilatation.

e **False** The urinary pH ranges from 4.8 to 7.5 and is usually less than 5.3. Manipulation of the pH of urine is occasionally used to aid the elimination of substances from the blood, for example forced alkaline diuresis in the treatment of salicylate poisoning and myoglobinuria.

Barrett K, Barman S, Boitano S, and Brooks HL (2009) *Ganong's Review of Medical Physiology*, 23rd edition. USA: McGraw-Hill.
Pinnock C, Lin T, and Smith T (2002) *Fundamentals of Anaesthesia*, 2nd edition. New York: Cambridge University Press.

27 Concerning white blood cells:

a **False** The normal range for the total white blood cell count is 4–11 × 10^9/l.

b **True** The neutrophils constitute approximately 40–75% of the total. Neutrophils are released in large quantities when bacteria invade the body. Neutrophils ingest the bacteria by phagocytosis and this is the first line of defence against infection.

c **True** The lymphocytes make up 20–45% of the total white cells. Most of lymphocytes are formed in the lymph nodes and only a few in the bone marrow.

d **True** Although they are few (between 2% and 6% of the total) in number, eosinophils are greatly increased in allergic conditions such as asthma or hay fever. These cells have antihistamine properties and congregate around sites of inflammation.

e **False** Monocytes make up 2–10% of the white cell count. They are phagocytic and invade areas of inflammation soon after neutrophils and help remove bacteria and debris. It is basophils which make up only 0.1% of the white cell count.

Allman K and Wilson I (2006) *Oxford Handbook of Anaesthesia*, 2nd edition. USA: Oxford University Press

Barrett K, Barman S, Boitano S, and Brooks HL (2009) *Ganong's Review of Medical Physiology*, 23rd edition. USA: McGraw-Hill.

28 Hypothermia:

a **True** Hypothermia is classed as a core body temperature less than 36°C. The National Institute for Health and Clinical Excellence has issued clinical guidelines in relation to inadvertent perioperative hypothermia which suggest that patients with a temperature of less than 36°C should be actively warmed prior to induction of anaesthesia.

b **True** Coagulation is impaired with hypothermia, as the enzymes involved in coagulation function optimally at body temperature. It is therefore important to warm blood administered during haemorrhage to avoid exacerbating the problem.

c **True** Vasoconstriction and increased viscosity of the blood both contribute to increased peripheral vascular resistance.

d **True** A temperature below 32°C predisposes to ventricular arrhythmia and at 28°C ventricular fibrillation occurs.

e **True** Hypothermia is used in situations where a complete circulatory arrest is necessary to perform complex heart surgery. It should be borne in mind that a hypothermic patient may need prolonged resuscitation as there are case reports of patients making complete recovery due to the protective effect of hypothermia reducing metabolism thus providing cerebral and cardiac protection.

Barrett K, Barman S, Boitano S, and Brooks HL (2009) *Ganong's Review of Medical Physiology*, 23rd edition. USA: McGraw-Hill.

National Institute for Health and Clinical Excellence. *Management of Inadvertent Perioperative Hypothermia in Adults*. Clinical guideline 65. London: National Institute for Health and Clinical Excellence. Available at: www.nice.org.uk.

29 Concerning renal function:

a **True** Plasma concentration of urea is 2.5–7 mmol/l and urine concentration is 200–400 mmol/l.

b **True** Normally the plasma urea:creatinine ratio is 10:1. The ratio is increased in prerenal uraemia from sodium and water depletion, cardiac failure, gastrointestinal haemorrhage, and trauma. Other causes include high protein intake, drugs impairing renal function, and protein catabolism, e.g. starvation and in the postoperative period.

c **True** If a substance has a smaller clearance than the glomerular filtration rate (GFR) then it must be reabsorbed, for example glucose. If clearance is greater than the GFR, the substance must be secreted by the renal tubules.

d **True** Inulin is a plant polysaccharide which is excreted by the kidneys in direct proportion to its plasma concentration over a very wide range. It is generally around 120–130 ml/min. In practice it is difficult to measure routinely. For this reason GFR is often calculated using the clearance of creatinine, or occasionally radiolabelled EDTA.

e **True** Under normal conditions all of the filtered glucose is reabsorbed. The majority of glucose reabsorption occurs in the proximal convoluted tubule, however, more distal parts of the nephron are capable of reabsorbing glucose. When the plasma glucose exceeds 11 mmol/l some nephrons exceed their capacity to reabsorb glucose and it becomes excreted in the urine.

Barrett K, Barman S, Boitano S, and Brooks HL (2009) *Ganong's Review of Medical Physiology*, 23rd edition. USA: McGraw-Hill.
Pinnock C, Lin T, and Smith T (2002) *Fundamentals of Anaesthesia*, 2nd edition. New York: Cambridge University Press.

30 Dopamine:

a **False** L-dopa or levodopa is a drug used in the treatment of Parkinson's disease and it is a precursor of dopamine. It is used as dopamine itself cannot cross the blood–brain barrier. Dopamine is a precursor of noradrenaline (norepinephrine) and adrenaline (epinephrine).

b **True** It is a neurotransmitter in the basal ganglia, it is involved with the integration of movement.

c **True** Insufficient levels of dopamine are responsible for the effects seen in Parkinson's disease. There is loss of dopamine in the striatum and substantia nigra. There is an imbalance between cholinergic and dopaminergic activity in the basal ganglia leading to abnormal movement. Treatment is aimed at increasing dopamine levels in the brain.

d **True** Dopamine in low dose infusion (less than 5 μg/kg/min) has previously been used for 'renal protection'. The dopamine increases blood flow to the kidneys via an increase in cardiac output and it is unlikely that there is a direct renal effect as previously thought.

e **True** It is secreted by the hypothalamus and inhibits prolactin.

Barrett K, Barman S, Boitano S, and Brooks HL (2009) *Ganong's Review of Medical Physiology*, 23rd edition. USA: McGraw-Hill.

chapter 4 PHARMACOLOGY

QUESTIONS

1 Codeine phosphate

a Is a prodrug of morphine
b Is naturally occurring
c Is not metabolized by up to 3% of the UK population
d May be used to increase the rate of intestinal transit
e Should not be given intramuscularly (IM)

2 Cyclizine:

a Is an antihistamine antiemetic
b Has an antimuscarinic action
c Has little effect against substances that act directly on the chemoreceptor trigger zone (CTZ)
d May produce dystonic reactions
e For intravenous (IV) administration has a pH of 6.8

3 Adrenergic receptor blocking drugs include:

a Labetalol
b Acebutolol
c Phenoxybenzamine
d Trimetaphan
e Clonidine

4 Trimetaphan:

a Is an adrenergic receptor blocking agent
b Has a longer duration of action than sodium nitroprusside
c Infusion should be preceded by IV atropine
d May lead to early tachyphylaxis during its use in younger patients
e Prolongs the action of suxamethonium

5 Heparin:

a Has a half-life of one to three hours
b Is basic
c In a dose of 100 units is equivalent to 10 mg
d May produce thrombocytopaenia
e Has a high lipid solubility

6 Salbutamol:

a Is a beta 1 adrenergic receptor agonist
b Is tocolytic
c Is available as a powder for inhalation
d May cause hyperglycaemia
e Is associated with hypokalaemia

7 Pethidine:

a Is more potent than morphine
b Has an atropine-like action
c Has a local anaesthetic action
d Is contraindicated in asthmatics
e Is safe to use in patients receiving monoamine oxidase inhibitors

8 Clonidine:

a Is an alpha 2 adrenergic receptor antagonist
b Has a central action
c Can be used to enhance caudal blocks
d Has no action on motor nerve fibres
e Has an oral bioavailability of almost 100%

9 Concerning benzodiazepines:

a They are anxiolytic neuroleptic agents
b They potentiate the action of analgesic drugs
c Midazolam is shorter acting than diazepam
d Diazepam has a half-life of 16 hours
e They may cause bronchospasm

10 Oxycodone:

a Is an opiate
b Is suitable for moderate to severe postoperative pain
c Is available in a short-acting form known as OxyContin
d Can cause arrhythmias
e May produce bronchospasm

11 Dantrolene sodium:

a Is a hydantoin derivative
b Can be used in the treatment of neuroleptic malignant syndrome
c In tablet form is used to treat chronic severe spasticity
d Potentiates non-depolarizing muscle relaxants
e Usual dose is 10 mg/kg every five minutes up to a maximum of 40 mg/kg in the acute management of malignant hyperpyrexia

12 Diamorphine:

a Is a natural alkaloid of opium
b Is also known as diacetylmorphine
c Crosses the blood–brain barrier more readily than morphine
d Produces analgesia lasting over eight hours when used in neuraxial blocks
e Has high oral bioavailability

13 Digoxin:

a Is derived from the foxglove plant
b Acts on the atrioventricular node to slow the ventricular rate
c Is a weak inotrope
d Therapeutic plasma levels are between 1 μg/l and 4 μg/l
e Has an elimination half-life of 18 hours

14 Suxamethonium:

a Produces dual block if repeated doses exceed 1 mg/kg
b Produces fasciculations in the eyelids and face first because these muscles are most sensitive to the drug
c Has a longer duration of action in malnutrition (e.g. kwashiorkor)
d Is hydrolysed in the neuromuscular junction
e Causes an increase in intragastric pressure

15 Desmopressin:

a Is a synthetic analogue of antidiuretic hormone (ADH)
b Has a similar vasopressor action to ADH
c Is used in diabetes insipidus
d Is contraindicated in haemophilia
e Has a half-life of three hours

16 Naloxone:

a Is a competitive antagonist of morphine
b Is given in a dose of 400–600 mg IV
c Is used to reverse narcotic-induced pruritus
d May cause pulmonary oedema
e Has a longer duration of action than morphine after intravenous administration

17 Droperidol:

a Is a butyrophenone derivative
b Antagonises D_2 receptors
c Is a weak antiemetic
d Has a duration of action lasting two hours
e Is contraindicated in Parkinson's disease

18 EMLA®:

a Is a eutectic mixture of local anaesthetics
b Contains lidocaine (lignocaine) 2.5% and prilocaine 5%
c Produces surface anaesthesia within 30 minutes
d May produce methaemoglobinaemia
e Maximum daily dose is 15 g or three tubes of cream

19 Esmolol:

a Is a cardioselective beta blocker
b Is metabolized by red cell esterases
c Is used for management of ventricular tachycardia
d Is available as an oral preparation
e Crosses the blood–brain barrier

20 Flumazenil:

a Is a benzodiazepine receptor antagonist
b Has a duration of action of 90 minutes
c May be given by infusion
d Is excreted unchanged in the urine
e Can precipitate seizures

21 Dopamine:

a Is a precursor of adrenaline (epinephrine)
b Has alpha 1 adrenergic, beta 1 adrenergic, and dopaminergic activity
c Deficiency leads to parkinsonism
d Suppresses growth hormone release
e Has a direct action on the CTZ and can cause nausea and vomiting

22 Glucagon:

a Is secreted by the beta cells of islets of Langerhans
b Mobilizes glycogen from the liver to raise blood sugar levels
c Has a hyperglycaemic action lasting for 100–120 minutes
d Is used in the treatment of beta blocker overdose
e Has a direct inotropic action

23 Papaverine:

a Is a smooth muscle relaxant
b Is a natural alkaloid of opium
c Is a direct vasodilator
d Is used in the management of intra-arterial thiopental (thiopentone) injection
e May be used to treat intestinal colic

24 Sodium nitroprusside:

- a Generates nitric oxide (NO) from the vessel wall to produce vasodilation
- b Has a greater action on preload than afterload
- c Is a long-acting hypotensive agent
- d Can produce cyanide ions and lactic acidosis if a total dose of 1.5 mg/kg is exceeded
- e Should be protected from light during administration

25 Mivacurium:

- a Has a duration of action between 25 and 35 minutes
- b Is usually administered in a dose of 0.07–0.25 mg/kg
- c Is hydrolysed by plasma cholinesterase
- d Has a vagolytic action
- e Causes significant histamine release

26 Ondansetron:

- a Is a H_1 receptor antagonist
- b Is available as IM, IV, oral, and rectal preparations
- c Prolongs the Q-T interval
- d Undergoes accelerated metabolism in patients treated with carbamazepine
- e May precipitate extrapyramidal signs

27 Side effects associated with the commonly used antiemetic drugs include:

- a Hypotension
- b Hypoxaemia
- c Oculogyric crisis
- d Tachycardia
- e Dry mouth

28 Phenytoin:

- a Is a hydantoin derivative
- b Is a class Ia antiarrhythmic
- c Has a half-life of 10 hours
- d Is 10% bound to protein in the blood
- e Is used in the treatment of all types of epilepsy

29 Oxytocin:

- a Is a posterior pituitary hormone
- b Causes uterine relaxation
- c Should be used with caution in cardiac disease
- d Has an antidiuretic action
- e May cause bradycardia

30 Rocuronium:

a Is an aminosteroid
b Is given in a dose of 0.6–1 mg/kg
c Is spontaneously hydrolysed in the blood
d Has a long duration of action of 60 minutes
e Is associated with significant histamine release

chapter 4 PHARMACOLOGY

ANSWERS

1 Codeine phosphate:

- a **True** Codeine is metabolized to morphine in the liver via the cytochrome P450 system (CYP2D6). It also has other metabolites, namely normorphine, norcodeine, and hydrocodone. Only morphine has an effect at mu receptors.
- b **True** Codeine occurs naturally and is otherwise known as methylmorhpine.
- c **False** Due to genetic polymorphism of the cytochrome P450 enzyme CYP2D6, approximately 5–10% of the UK population are poor metabolizers of codeine, therefore reducing the analgesic benefit of the drug.
- d **True** Codeine is used in chronic diarrhoea to increase the transit time in the gastrointestinal tract.
- e **False** Codeine should not be administered intravenously as it is associated with hypotension which may be caused by histamine release. This effect is not seen with the oral or IM routes, which are safe.

Peck T, Hill S, and Williams M (2004) *Pharmacology for Anaesthesia and Intensive Care*, 2nd edition. Cambridge: Cambridge University Press.

Yentis S, Hirsh N, and Smith G (2003) *Anaesthesia and Intensive Care A to Z*, 3rd edition. London: Butterworth-Heinemann.

2 Cyclizine:

- a **True** Cyclizine is a piperazine derivative. It is a histamine (H_1) receptor antagonist and also has anticholinergic properties.
- b **True** Hence it produces tachycardia.
- c **True** It is more effective against nausea and vomiting caused by labyrinthine disorders and travel sickness.
- d **False** Dystonic reactions are seen with antidopaminergic drugs, e.g. metoclopramide, prochlorperazine, and perphenazine.
- e **False** It has a pH of 3.2 as it is prepared with lactic acid and is therefore painful when given IV or IM.

Allman K and Wilson I (2006) *Oxford Handbook of Anaesthesia*, 2nd edition. New York: Oxford University Press.

Peck T, Hill S, and Williams M (2004) *Pharmacology for Anaesthesia and Intensive Care*, 2nd edition. Cambridge: Cambridge University Press.

3 Adrenergic receptor blocking drugs include:

a **True** Labetalol is an alpha and beta blocker and is one of the drugs used for providing controlled hypotension during anaesthesia.

b **True** It is a beta blocker with intrinsic sympathomimetic activity (ISA), or a cardioselective beta blocker. It is only available orally.

c **True** It is a long-acting alpha blocker (half-life 24 hours) and hence used in specific situations only, such as preoperative preparation for surgical management of phaeochromocytoma.

d **False** It is a ganglion blocker, antagonizing nicotinic receptors at sympathetic and parasympathetic ganglia. It has been used extensively in the past for controlled hypotension, before drugs such as sodium nitroprusside were available. It is one of the drugs which will prolong the action of suxamethonium by inhibiting plasma cholinesterase.

e **False** It is an alpha 2 agonist used to treat hypertension, acute and chronic pain, and for sedation in intensive care.

Table 4.1 Summary of adrenergic receptors

Agonist	Phenylephrine	Clonidine			
	Methoxamine	α-methyl noradrenaline			
			Dobutamine	Terbutaline	
	Noradrenaline			Salbutamol	Noradrenaline
	Adrenaline				
			Isoprenaline		
Receptors	α_1 Vascular	α_2 Presynaptic	β_1 Heart	β_2 Smooth	β_3 Fat
Antagonists	Labetolol		Labetolol		CGP20712A
	Phentolamine		Propranolol		
	Phenoxybenzamine		Atenolol	Butoxamine	
	Prazosin	Yohombine	Metoprolol		
Potencies	A = NA » Iso	A = NA » Iso	Iso > A = NA	Iso > A » NA	Iso = NA > A

A, adrenaline; NA, noradrenaline; Iso, isoprenaline.

Peck T, Hill S, and Williams M (2004) *Pharmacology for Anaesthesia and Intensive Care*, 2nd edition. Cambridge: Cambridge University Press.

4 Trimetaphan:

a **False** It antagonizes nicotinic receptors at both parasympathetic and sympathetic ganglia, and the adrenal cortex.
b **True** Although the hypotensive effects have the same duration as those of nitroprusside, the other ganglion-blocking effects, e.g. dilation of the pupils, may last several hours after discontinuing a trimetaphan infusion.
c **False** Any drug that is likely to increase heart rate should be avoided prior to the use of trimetaphan for controlled hypotension as the hypotension is accompanied by a compensatory tachycardia.
d **True** The autonomic response to hypotension is reflex tachycardia, which is much more active in young patients. The tachycardia aims to negate the hypotensive effect of the drug and hence the tachyphylaxis.
e **True** It is one of the drugs known to prolong the action of suxamethonium as it inhibits plasma cholinesterase.

Allman K and Wilson I (2006) *Oxford Handbook of Anaesthesia*, 2nd edition. New York: Oxford University Press.

5 Heparin:

a **True** Given intravenously it has a half-life of one to three hours.
b **False** Heparin is an anionic, mucopolysaccharide organic acid.
c **False** 1 mg of heparin is equal to 100 units. In open heart surgery a dose of 3 mg (300 units)/kg is commonly used as the loading dose, i.e. 21 000 units.
d **True** This is a type II immune-mediated reaction occurring after four to 14 days of administration of either fractionated or unfractionated heparin. Heparin causes platelet aggregation and arterial and venous thromboses.
e **False** Heparin is charged, has high protein binding and a low lipid solubility, and does not cross the blood–brain barrier or the placenta.

Allman K and Wilson I (2006) *Oxford Handbook of Anaesthesia*, 2nd edition. New York: Oxford University Press.

6 Salbutamol:

a **False** It is a beta 2 agonist and hence a more selective bronchodilator.
b **True** It relaxes the gravid uterus and has been used occasionally in premature labour.
c **True** The dry powder is available in doses of 200–400 µg in capsules for inhalation, or as a 100 µg metered-dose inhaler for use in chronic asthma.
d **True** Salbutamol may increase blood sugar levels particularly when corticosteroids are co-administered. It should be used with caution in diabetes, especially when given IV due to the risk of precipitating diabetic ketoacidosis.
e **True** Dangerous hypokalaemia may occur with high doses of beta 2 agonist, especially in the acute situation where the patient may also be receiving theophylline, corticosteroids, and diuretics, all of which will potentiate any hypokalaemia.

Allman K and Wilson I (2006) *Oxford Handbook of Anaesthesia*, 2nd edition. New York: Oxford University Press.

7 Pethidine:

a **False** Pethidine has only one-tenth of the potency of morphine and is not suitable for severe continuing pain.

b **True** In addition to its analgesic actions it also has anticholinergic actions. Tachycardia used to be a problem when was given as premedication along with atropine.

c **True** Pethidine also has a local anaesthetic action. Preservative-free pethidine has been used as a sole agent in spinal anaesthesia in the past; however, its widespread use is limited by the increased levels of nausea and vomiting it produces compared with other agents.

d **False** It is a safe drug to use in asthmatic patients. It causes a small amount of histamine release, but also causes bronchodilation.

e **False** Pethidine should be avoided in patients on monoamine oxidase inhibitors. When these drugs are co-administered there is an increase in central 5-HT activity leading to agitation, hypertension, tachycardia, pyrexia, convulsions and coma.

Peck T, Hill S, and Williams M (2004) *Pharmacology for Anaesthesia and Intensive Care*, 2nd edition. Cambridge: Cambridge University Press.
Yentis S, Hirsh N, and Smith G (2003) *Anaesthesia and Intensive Care A to Z*, 3rd edition. London: Butterworth-Heinemann.

8 Clonidine:

a **False** Clonidine is an alpha receptor agonist with 200 times more affinity for alpha 2 than alpha 1 receptors. Stimulation of presynaptic alpha 2 receptors causes a suppression of catecholamine release by negative feedback control.

b **True** It acts at the lateral reticular nucleus to reduce central sympathetic outflow. It also acts at spinal cord level to enhance endorphin release, with an opioid-sparing effect and to enhance descending inhibitory pathways involved in perception of pain.

c **True** Clonidine can be added to the local anaesthetic used in both paediatric and adult caudal blocks to increase the duration of action. It can also be used via the subarachnoid route. Unlike opioids it is not associated with respiratory depression, making it safe to use even in day-case anaesthesia.

d **True** It prolongs blocks when given in addition to local anaesthetics, but does not produce motor or sensory blockade itself.

e **True** For this reason it is effective in tablet form and is used in doses of 150–300 μg, up to a maximum of 1.2 g/day. It is used in chronic pain and also in opioid and alcohol withdrawal for its anxiolytic properties.

Allman K and Wilson I (2006) *Oxford Handbook of Anaesthesia*, 2nd edition. New York: Oxford University Press.
Peck T, Hill S, and Williams M (2004) *Pharmacology for Anaesthesia and Intensive Care*, 2nd edition. Cambridge: Cambridge University Press.

9 Concerning benzodiazepines:

a **False** They are anxiolytics and not neuroleptics.

b **False** They have no analgesic action and do not therefore potentiate analgesics.

c **True** The duration of action is 20–60 minutes only due to distribution.

d **False** It has a half-life of between 20 and 40 hours, it has the lowest clearance of all of the benzodiazepines.

e **False** Respiratory depression is seen with benzodiazepines and not bronchospasm.

Allman K and Wilson I (2006) *Oxford Handbook of Anaesthesia*, 2nd edition. New York: Oxford University Press.
Rang H, Dale M, and Ritter J (2000) *Rang and Dales' Pharmacology*, 6th edition. Edinburgh: Churchill Livingstone.

10 Oxycodone:

a **False** It is an opioid derivative of morphine.
b **True** Its main use, however, lies in the management of chronic pain, especially in palliative care.
c **False** OxyContin is a long-acting version of oxycodone and is prescribed in a single dose of 20 mg daily in adults.
d **True** It may produce supraventricular tachycardia.
e **True** Like other opioids it can produce respiratory depression and may also cause bronchospasm secondary to histamine release.

Allman K and Wilson I (2006) *Oxford Handbook of Anaesthesia*, 2nd edition. New York: Oxford University Press.
British National Formulary 59 (2009) Chapter 4.7.2: Opioid analgesics. London: BMJ Group and RPS Publishing.

11 Dantrolene sodium:

a **True** It has a similar structure to phenytoin. It acts by inhibiting release of calcium ions from the sarcoplasmic reticulum in striated muscle thereby uncoupling the excitation–contraction process.
b **True** Management of neuroleptic malignant syndrome is essentially supportive, although active cooling, bromocriptine, and dantrolene have also been used.
c **True** The oral dose of 25 mg daily can be increased up to 100 mg four times daily in adults.
d **True** Since it is a direct acting muscle relaxant, it potentiates other drugs with similar actions.
e **False** The initial dose is 2–3 mg/kg, which may be repeated to a maximum of 10 mg/kg.

Allman K and Wilson I (2006) *Oxford Handbook of Anaesthesia*, 2nd edition. New York: Oxford University Press.
Association of Anaesthetists of Great Britain and Ireland (2007) *Guidelines for the Management of a Malignant Hyperthermia Crisis*. London: Association of Anaesthetists of Great Britain and Ireland.

12 Diamorphine:

a **False** It is a purified extract of morphine, with no affinity for opioid receptors. It is a prodrug of morphine, being 1.5 to two times as potent. All of its effects are via its metabolites.
b **True** It is also known as heroin.
c **True** Hence the heightened feeling of well being compared to morphine, making it much more addictive.
d **True** 0.25–0.5 mg used in spinal anaesthesia can give analgesia over 10–12 hours. The possibility of late-onset respiratory depression exists if other narcotic agents are co-administered.
e **False** Diamorphine has high lipid solubility and is therefore well absorbed from the gut. However, it undergoes extensive first-pass metabolism, which means it has low oral bioavailability. It is therefore mainly given via parenteral routes although it is available in tablet form.

Allman K and Wilson I (2006) *Oxford Handbook of Anaesthesia*, 2nd edition. New York: Oxford University Press.
British National Formulary 59 (2009) Chapter 4.7.2: Opioid analgesics. London: BMJ Group and RPS Publishing.

13 Digoxin:

a **True** It is a glycoside, extracted from the leaves of *Digitalis lanata* (foxglove). It inhibits cardiac sodium/potassium ATPase, producing an increased intracellular sodium ion concentration and a decrease in intracellular potassium ions. The increase in intracellular sodium ions allows more exchange of intracellular sodium for extracellular calcium ions. The increase in intracellular calcium ions increases the force of cardiac contraction. It also leads to increased cardiac muscarinic receptor acetylcholine, which slows conduction at the atrioventricular node and bundle of His.

b **True** It is used in the treatment of atrial fibrillation and flutter for this effect. By slowing the ventricular rate the heart can function more efficiently by lengthening diastole, thus improving coronary perfusion.

c **True** It is better at controlling heart rate than increasing the contractility.

d **False** Its therapeutic ratio is very narrow, 0.5–2 μg/l. Side effects are common and are enhanced by hypokalaemia.

e **False** The elimination half life is approximately 35 hours in patients with normal renal function and is much more prolonged in renal impairment, requiring dose reduction.

Allman K and Wilson I (2006) *Oxford Handbook of Anaesthesia*, 2nd edition. New York: Oxford University Press.

Peck T, Hill S, and Williams M (2004) *Pharmacology for Anaesthesia and Intensive Care*, 2nd edition. Cambridge: Cambridge University Press.

14 Suxamethonium:

a **False** Dual block, or phase II block, may be seen if the dosage exceeds 400–500 mg as an infusion or repeated doses. Build up of succinyl monocholine, a breakdown product of hydrolysis, has a weak non-depolarizing relaxant effect, which is considered responsible for the dual block. It is more commonly seen in myasthenia gravis and with the concurrent use of acetylcholinesterase inhibitors.

b **False** The drug reaches the head and neck before the trunk and lower body because of the short distance from the heart, and hence the fasciculations appear in the face first.

c **True** One of the acquired causes of pseudocholinesterase deficiency is malnutrition and the inability of the liver produce the enzyme. Pregnancy, burns, plasmapheresis, and protein deficiency are other causes of reduced pseudocholinesterase.

d **False** Suxamethonium is hydrolysed by pseudocholinesterase or plasma cholinesterase, which is not present in the neuromuscular junction. This is the reason why the action of suxamethonium is longer than the action of acetylcholine at the neuromuscular junction.

e **True** There is an increase in intragastric pressure by approximately 10 mmHg. This effect increases the risk of pulmonary aspiration of gastric contents, however, it is offset by a simultaneous increase in lower oesophageal sphincter pressure.

Allman K and Wilson I (2006) *Oxford Handbook of Anaesthesia*, 2nd edition. New York: Oxford University Press.

Yentis S, Hirsh N, and Smith G (2003) *Anaesthesia and Intensive Care A to Z*, 3rd edition. London: Butterworth-Heinemann.

15 Desmopressin:

a **True** D-deamino-8-D-arginine-vasopressin is an analogue of vasopressin (arginine vasopressin (AVP), or ADH).
b **False** It is longer acting than ADH but has less vasopressor action.
c **True** It is particularly useful in the management of neurogenic diabetes insipidus, where it can be administered orally, IV or intranasally.
d **False** Desmopressin enhances factor VIII activity and is used to increase levels of factor VIII by two to four times in haemophilia and von Willebrand's disease.
e **False** Its half-life is 75 minutes.

Peck T, Hill S, and Williams M (2004) *Pharmacology for Anaesthesia and Intensive Care*, 2nd edition. Cambridge: Cambridge University Press.
Yentis S, Hirsh N, and Smith G (2003) *Anaesthesia and Intensive Care A to Z*, 3rd edition. London: Butterworth-Heinemann.

16 Naloxone:

a **True** Naloxone is a pure opioid antagonist. It has an affinity for all the opioid receptors but with a higher affinity for mu receptors.
b **False** It is administered in a dose of 100–400 μg, titrated to effect.
c **True** Troublesome pruritus is associated with opioid administration, especially intrathecal opioids. Antihistamines do not help relieve the pruritus. Naloxone as a bolus followed by an infusion is effective.
d **True** Administration, particularly with a rapid IV bolus, may cause hypertension, pulmonary oedema, and cardiac arrhythmias.
e **False** The duration of action of naloxone, 30–40 minutes, is shorter than that of morphine, and so an infusion may be required to avoid re-narcotization.

Allman K and Wilson I (2006) *Oxford Handbook of Anaesthesia*, 2nd edition. New York: Oxford University Press.

17 Droperidol:

a **True** Of the dopamine antagonists, droperidol was the only butyrophenone, but it is no longer used.
b **True** Droperidol acts as an antagonist at the D_2 receptors in the CTZ to prevent nausea and vomiting.
c **False** It is a potent antiemetic with a long duration of action.
d **False** Its action lasts for up to four hours.
e **True** It is known to cause extrapyramidal effects and should be avoided in Parkinson's disease.

Allman K and Wilson I (2006) *Oxford Handbook of Anaesthesia*, 2nd edition. New York: Oxford University Press.
Peck T, Hill S, and Williams M (2004) *Pharmacology for Anaesthesia and Intensive Care*, 2nd edition. Cambridge: Cambridge University Press.

18 EMLA®:

a **True** When mixed together in equal quantities by weight the local anaesthetics form a 'eutectic mixture' in which the melting point is lower than its individual components.

b **False** It contains equal quantities of lidocaine (lignocaine) 2.5% and prilocaine 2.5% as an oil–water emulsion. EMLA® cream has a melting point of 16°C.

c **False** It requires 60–90 minutes to produce satisfactory anaesthesia.

d **True** Since it contains prilocaine, increases in methaemoglobin may be produced after large doses. However, the blood levels reached after a standard application are too low to encounter it.

e **False** It is used by some for taking split skin grafts from a wide area. The maximum dose is 60 g or 12 tubes of 5 g each or two tubes of 30 g each (available as a surgical pack).

Allman K and Wilson I (2006) *Oxford Handbook of Anaesthesia*, 2nd edition. New York: Oxford University Press.

British National Formulary 59 (2009) Chapter 15.2: Local anaesthesia. London: BMJ Group and RPS Publishing.

19 Esmolol:

a **True** Other cardioselective beta blockers include metoprolol, atenolol, and acebutolol.

b **True** This accounts for its short half-life of about 10 minutes. It is metabolized to inactive metabolites.

c **False** Its main indication is for the treatment supraventricular tachycardia. It is also used for the management of intraoperative hypertension and tachycardia.

d **False** Esmolol is only available for IV use. It is diluted and administered as an infusion or as boluses titrated to effect.

e **True** Esmolol is highly lipid soluble, and therefore it is able to cross the blood–brain barrier to produce sedation and nightmares.

Allman K and Wilson I (2006) *Oxford Handbook of Anaesthesia*, 2nd edition. New York: Oxford University Press.

Peck T, Hill S, and Williams M (2004) *Pharmacology for Anaesthesia and Intensive Care*, 2nd edition. Cambridge: Cambridge University Press.

20 Flumazenil:

a **True** It is a competitive antagonist used to reverse the effects of benzodiazepines. It does not affect the metabolism of benzodiazepines.

b **False** It has a relatively short duration of action of approximately 60 minutes.

c **True** As flumazenil has a short duration of action its effects may wear off before the effects of the benzodiazepine so an infusion may be required. A dose of 100–400 μg/h is used.

d **False** A significant proportion of the drug undergoes hepatic metabolism to inactive metabolites and is excreted in the urine.

e **True** Seizures can occur if flumazenil is given to patients on long-term benzodiazepines, for example, patients with epilepsy.

Allman K and Wilson I (2006) *Oxford Handbook of Anaesthesia*, 2nd edition. New York: Oxford University Press.

Peck T, Hill S, and Williams M (2004) *Pharmacology for Anaesthesia and Intensive Care*, 2nd edition. Cambridge: Cambridge University Press.

21 Dopamine:

a **False** It is a precursor of noradrenaline (norepinephrine).

b **True** The effects at each receptor depends on the dose of dopamine. Up to 5 μg/kg/min dopamine receptor stimulation causes renal and mesenteric vasodilation, increasing blood flow. Between 5 μg/kg/min and 15 μg/kg/min beta 1 adrenergic receptor stimulation occurs, increasing cardiac output via an increase in heart rate and contractility. Over 15 μg/kg/min, alpha 1 adrenergic receptor stimulation leads to peripheral vasoconstriction.

c **True** Dopamine is a central neurotransmitter in the basal ganglia and deficiency leads to the various symptoms of parkinsonism.

d **True** Dopamine suppresses the release of oxytocin and other pituitary hormones.

e **True** Some antiemetics have antidopaminergic action, e.g. metoclopramide and prochlorperazine.

Allman K and Wilson I (2006) *Oxford Handbook of Anaesthesia*, 2nd edition. New York: Oxford University Press.

Peck T, Hill S, and Williams M (2004) *Pharmacology for Anaesthesia and Intensive Care*, 2nd edition. Cambridge: Cambridge University Press.

22 Glucagon:

a **False** It is a polypeptide hormone secreted from the alpha cells of the islets of Langerhans.

b **True** When glucagon is administered to a hypoglycaemic patient, the blood sugar is rapidly increased. A dextrose infusion may also be required.

c **False** The hyperglycaemic action lasts only 10–30 minutes and hence the need for the dextrose infusion to be started simultaneously.

d **True** It stimulates adenyl cyclase and consequently its actions are similar to the beta adrenoceptor activity of adrenaline (epinephrine) and helps overcome the effects of beta blockers. It is usually necessary to administer glucagon as an infusion due to its short duration of action.

e **True** It is not as potent as adrenaline.

Peck T, Hill S, and Williams M (2004) *Pharmacology for Anaesthesia and Intensive Care*, 2nd edition. Cambridge: Cambridge University Press.

23 Papaverine:

a **True** Papaverine is believed to block calcium channels in addition to phosphodiesterase (PDE) inhibition, producing relaxation of the smooth muscle of vessels. Other PDE inhibitors include the methylxanthines, e.g. theophylline, which produce relaxation of non-vascular smooth muscle, namely bronchial muscle. Aminophylline, which is a theophylline derivative, has also been used for this purpose.

b **True** Structurally it is a benzylisoquinoline opium alkaloid. It is found with morphine in opium, but despite this it has no analgesic properties.

c **True** The exact mechanism of action is unclear. Papaverine's non-specific relaxant effect on smooth muscle is used in vascular surgery. It is available in a 40 mg/ml ampoule, which is diluted to 20 ml and given slowly IV.

d **True** Papaverine may be used for its direct action on vascular smooth muscle to reduce the arterial spasm seen with accidental injection of thiopental (thiopentone).

e **True** It is used in combination oral preparations to relieve gastrointestinal smooth muscle spasm.

Peck T, Hill S, and Williams M (2004) *Pharmacology for Anaesthesia and Intensive Care*, 2nd edition. Cambridge: Cambridge University Press.

Yentis S, Hirsh N, and Smith G (2003) *Anaesthesia and Intensive Care A to Z*, 3rd edition. London: Butterworth-Heinemann.

24 Sodium nitroprusside:

a **True** Sodium nitroprusside is an inorganic complex that acts as a prodrug. It reacts with tissue sulphydryl groups to produce nitric oxide, which activates guanylate cyclase increasing intracellular cyclic guanosine monophosphate (GMP) and decreasing cytoplasmic calcium, thus relaxing smooth muscle and producing vasodilation.

b **False** It has equal action on arterial and venous smooth muscle. Arterial vasodilation reduces the systemic venous resistance (SVR), thus reducing the blood pressure and afterload. Venous vasodilation reduces the preload by increasing the venous capacitance.

c **False** It has on onset within three minutes and is rapidly broken down so that is has a short half-life with a duration of action of less than 10 minutes.

d **True** Usual dosage during anaesthesia is 0.3–1.5 μg/kg/min. If the total dose infused exceeds 1.5 mg/kg, there is a risk of cyanide poisoning.

e **True** Exposure to light hydrolyses nitroprusside to cyanide and hence the need to cover the bag and the infusion set with reflective aluminium foil or consider use of opaque syringes and giving sets.

Peck T, Hill S, and Williams M (2004) *Pharmacology for Anaesthesia and Intensive Care*, 2nd edition. Cambridge: Cambridge University Press.

Yentis S, Hirsh N, and Smith G (2003) *Anaesthesia and Intensive Care A to Z*, 3rd edition. London: Butterworth-Heinemann.

25 Mivacurium:

a **False** It is short acting and its effect only lasts between 10 and 20 minutes.
b **True** This is the intubation dose. Bigger doses increase the duration of action and hence a 0.25 mg/kg dose lasts approximately 23 minutes.
c **True** In patients with deficiency of this enzyme due to genetic polymorphism or in liver disease, its action may be considerably prolonged. A proportion of the drug is metabolized by the liver.
d **False** It does not have any action on the vagus. High doses are associated with a decrease in blood pressure secondary to histamine release.
e **True** For this reason mivacurium use is avoided in asthmatic patients.

Allman K and Wilson I (2006) *Oxford Handbook of Anaesthesia*, 2nd edition. New York: Oxford University Press.

26 Ondansetron:

a **False** It is a selective serotonin (5-hydroxytryptamine$_3$) receptor antagonist.
b **True** The different formulations make it extremely versatile for use across a range of ages. Per rectum use is associated with rectal irritation.
c **True** Ondansetron can prolong the Q-T interval and lead to heart block. It is therefore best avoided in patients prone to arrhythmias.
d **True** Carbamazepine and phenytoin both lead to increased metabolism of ondansetron and reduced efficacy.
e **True** Although not as common as with metoclopramide, extrapyramidal side effects have been reported with the use of ondansetron.

Allman K and Wilson I (2006) *Oxford Handbook of Anaesthesia*, 2nd edition. New York: Oxford University Press.
British National Formulary 59 (2009) Chapter 4.6 Drugs used in the treatment of nausea and vertigo. London: BMJ Group and RPS Publishing.

27 Side effects associated with the commonly used antiemetic drugs include:

a **False** In the past, phenothiazines were mainly responsible for hypotension. Prochlorperazine (Stemetil), which is the only phenothiazine in common use presently, does not cause the same degree of hypotension as others in this group, e.g. chlorpromazine and perphenazine.
b **False** Hypoxaemia does not occur, although the drugs can cause drowsiness.
c **True** Metoclopramide causes extrapyramidal reactions, especially in females and young patients. There are a few reports of ondansetron also causing extrapyramidal reactions.
d **True** Cyclizine, which has an anticholinergic action, may be responsible for tachycardia, especially after IV administration.
e **True** This is an anticholinergic response.

Table 4.2 Drugs commonly used in postoperative nausea and vomiting

Class of agent	Drug	Dose	Comments	Problems
Antimuscarinic	Hyoscine	0.4 mg	Effective as premedicant	Sedative; central anticholinergic syndrome
Antihistamine	Cyclizine	50 mg		Antimuscarinic effects, heart failure after MI, sedation
Antidopaminergic (procainamide derivative)	Metoclopramide	(10 mg) 25–50 mg	Questionable efficacy, may need higher dose	EP side effects
Antidopaminergic (piperazine phenothiazine)	Prochlorperazine	5–12.5 mg	No IV preparation	EP, hypotension, neuroleptic malignant syndrome
Antidopaminergic (butyrophenone)	Droperidol	<1 mg	Effective at low doses, comparable with $5HT_3$ blockers	Not likely at low doses; withdrawn in UK because of concerns about dysrhythmia (Q-T prologation etc.)
$5HT_3$ antagonists	Ondansetron Also: Granisetron Tropisetron Dolasetron	4–8 mg 1–3 mg 2–5 mg Up to 12.5 mg	NNT 4–7 Higher dose may be more effective	Adverse effects uncommon (headache, constipation, raised liver enzymes)
Corticosteroids	Dexamethasone	2.5–8 mg	NNT 4 Unknown mechanism	Not likely with very short-term use; can cause perineal burning sensation in awake patient

5HT, 5-hydroxytryptamine; IV, intravenous; NNT, numbers needed to treat; EP, extrapyramidal.

Aitkenhead A and Smith G (2008) *Textbook of Anaesthesia*, 5th edition. Edinburgh: Churchill Livingstone.
Kevin K and Spoors C (2009) *Training in Anaesthesia*. New York: Oxford University Press.

28 Phenytoin:

a **True** Phenytoin, like dantrolene, is a hydantoin derivative. Its main uses are in the treatment of epilepsy and chronic pain.

b **False** It is a class Ib antiarrhythmic with a membrane stabilizing effect. It acts at the sodium channel to shorten the length of the refractory period of cardiac muscle.

c **False** It is greater than 20–24 hours. Elimination follows first order kinetics until plasma levels exceed 10 mg/l when zero order kinetics occur due to saturation of enzyme systems.

d **False** Approximately 90% is bound to albumin.

e **False** It is not used in the treatment of petit mal epilepsy.

Allman K and Wilson I (2006) *Oxford Handbook of Anaesthesia*, 2nd edition. New York: Oxford University Press.
Peck T, Hill S, and Williams M (2004) *Pharmacology for Anaesthesia and Intensive Care*, 2nd edition. Cambridge: Cambridge University Press.

29 Oxytocin:

a **True** ADH (vasopressin) is another posterior pituitary hormone.

b **False** Oxytocin causes smooth muscle contraction in the uterus and the milk ducts. It is used in labour to augment uterine contractions and to aid delivery of the placenta and contraction of the uterus to prevent post-partum haemorrhage.

c **True** It is associated with severe hypotension when administered to patients with cardiac disease. Oxytocin causes a transient reduction in SVR and BP while the autotransfusion of blood from the contracting uterus causes a sudden increase in central venous pressure. ST depression during administration has been reported even in patients with no cardiac disease.

d **True** It has a modest antidiuretic action and may cause water retention. Severe hyponatraemia has been caused by administration of oxytocin diluted with dextrose solutions.

e **False** Tachycardia is associated with its use, especially when administered as a rapid IV bolus.

Allman K and Wilson I (2006) *Oxford Handbook of Anaesthesia*, 2nd edition. New York: Oxford University Press.
Peck T, Hill S, and Williams M (2004) *Pharmacology for Anaesthesia and Intensive Care*, 2nd edition. Cambridge: Cambridge University Press.

30 Rocuronium:

a **True** It is an aminosteroid, non-depolarizing muscle relaxant developed from vecuronium. It has a quicker onset than vecuronium.

b **True** When given in a dose of 1 mg/kg, rocuronium has a rapid onset of around 45 seconds to one minute, making it a suitable alternative to use in a modified rapid sequence induction when suxamethonium is contraindicated.

c **False** It is partly metabolized and partly excreted unchanged in bile and urine. It does not undergo spontaneous hydrolysis meaning it requires reversal. Concerns over its duration of action when used in a modified rapid sequence may be allayed by the introduction of the novel reversal agent sugammadex. During routine use, rocuronium is reversed with neostigmine.

d **False** It has a medium duration of action of up to 40 minutes.

e **False** It is not associated with histamine release and is safe to use in asthmatic patients as an alternative to atracurium, which does cause histamine release.

Allman K and Wilson I (2006) *Oxford Handbook of Anaesthesia*, 2nd edition. New York: Oxford University Press.
Peck T, Hill S, and Williams M (2004) *Pharmacology for Anaesthesia and Intensive Care*, 2nd edition. Cambridge: Cambridge University Press.

chapter 4

PHYSICS

QUESTIONS

1 During invasive arterial pressure monitoring:

a A rigid cannula must be used
b The tubing connecting the cannula to the transducer should not be longer than 1 m
c The tubing is connected to a soft diaphragm consisting of a Wheatstone bridge circuit
d Pulse pressure can be ascertained
e The system used to measure the pressure should be capable of responding to a frequency range of 0.45–40 Hz

2 The pneumotachograph:

a Is a device used for measuring gas flow
b Is unidirectional
c Has a fixed resistance with pressure transducers across it measuring the pressure drop
d The flow pattern is laminar through the resistance
e Water vapour condensation at the resistance can cause inaccuracies

3 Concerning ventilator alarms:

a They can be pressure or volume monitoring alarms
b Pressure alarm monitors are fitted on the expiratory limb
c Volume alarm monitors need either a respirometer or a pneumotachograph to measure the gas flow.
d Volume alarms are fitted on to the inspiratory limb
e Both pressure and volume alarms are mandatory to detect disconnection or obstruction in the ventilator circuit.

4 Regarding peripheral nerve stimulators:

a The negative electrode is placed over the proximal nerve and the positive electrode is placed over the most superficial part of the nerve
b They deliver a variable current at the nerve
c Train-of-four is the ratio of the fourth twitch height to that of the first
d 150–200 Hz is used in tetanic stimulation
e In double-burst stimulation, two short bursts of 100 Hz are applied with a 750 ms interval

5 Tympanic membrane temperature:

a Is commonly measured using an infrared thermometer
b Correlates well with brain temperature
c Is lower than the core temperature as measured in the oesophagus
d Can be measured with a thermocouple or a thermistor probe
e Is as accurate as the bladder temperature in an anaesthetized patient

6 Nerve stimulators used for nerve blocks:

a Have two leads—the negative lead is attached to the skin and the positive lead to the needle
b Deliver a stimulus for 100–200 ms
c Usually use a frequency of 1–2 Hz
d Can be substituted with peripheral nerve stimulators used for monitoring neuromuscular blockade
e Assist in producing a successful block if muscular twitch is seen to disappear at a current of 0.4 mA

7 Continuous positive airway pressure (CPAP):

a Refers to positive pressure applied to a spontaneously breathing patient
b Should be applied at 5–25 cmH_2O for efficient results
c May reduce cardiac output
d Can be delivered more efficiently using a nasal mask than a face mask
e Is more efficient than invasive positive pressure ventilation (IPPV) in hyaline membrane disease of the newborn

8 Flow through intravenous cannulae:

a 22 G 15–20 ml/min
b 20 G 30–40 ml/min
c 18 G 60–80 ml/min
d 16 G 120–200 ml/min
e 14 G 250–360 ml/min

9 Concerning intravenous (IV) administration of fluids:

a Adult giving sets have an internal diameter of 6 mm
b A blood filter has a mesh size of 75 μm
c There are 15 drops of crystalloid fluid per ml with an adult giving set
d There are 30 drops of crystalloid fluid per ml in a paediatric giving set
e A burette with a drop size of 15 drops per ml can used for paediatric blood transfusion.

10 The pH electrode:

a Measures the hydrogen ions in a sample
b Can be used for measuring the pH of blood and urine
c Has a mercury/mercury chloride measuring electrode and a silver/silver chloride reference electrode
d Measures the electrical potential that is created as a result of the pH gradient between the two electrodes
e A linear electrical output of about 0.6 mV per unit of pH is produced

11 Defibrillators:

a Deliver alternating current
b Possess an inductor that discharges current from the machine to the patient
c Have external paddles, one of which can be placed over the precordium and the other positioned posteriorly behind the heart
d Release electrical energy that is dissipated throughout the skin and tissues with only about 35 amps reaching the heart
e Deliver a shock synchronized with the T wave of the electrocardiogram (ECG) to treat ventricular arrhythmias

12 Maintenance measures for gas cylinders include:

a Storage in an upright position
b Covering the valve outlets with grease during storage
c Storage in a cold place
d The manufacturer performing periodic 'hydraulic stretch tests'
e Not exceeding a filling ratio of 0.69 for nitrous oxide cylinders

13 With regard to lasers:

a The acronym 'laser' stands for light augmentation by the simultaneous emission of radiation
b Carbon dioxide lasers are used for ophthalmic surgery
c When used in ENT surgery, lasers require a special endotracheal tube to be used
d When used in an intubated patient, lasers require the endotracheal cuff to be inflated with saline instead of air
e They can cause permanent damage to the retina or the optic nerve of theatre personnel if suitable protection is not worn

14 Regarding latex and latex allergy:

a Latex is a natural substance
b Latex allergy is more common in people who have an allergy to certain foods including avocado, banana, and chestnut
c RAST may be used in latex allergy diagnosis
d The majority of anaesthetic equipment used in theatres is latex free
e Rubber stoppers should be removed from vials before drawing up drugs in a latex allergy case

15 Regarding epidural needles:

a The standard epidural needle in use is 14 G and 10 cm long
b It has a bevel at an angle of 5° to the shaft with a blunt leading edge
c The bevel is known as the 'Huber point'
d A 20 cm long version is available for obese patients
e A 19 G needle is available for use in paediatrics

16 Epidural catheters:

- a Are 60 cm long
- b Have an external diameter of 2 mm and an internal diameter of 1 mm
- c May be radio-opaque to check the accuracy of positioning
- d Should not be withdrawn through the Tuohy needle once threaded through the bevel
- e Have a filter of 0.22 μm mesh size through which drugs are injected

17 Concerning spinal needles:

- a The most commonly used size for intrathecal anaesthesia is 21 G
- b They are usually 18 cm long
- c They are usually passed through an 18 G or 19 G introducer needle
- d The cutting point type are associated with more postdural puncture headaches than the pencil point type
- e The Whitacre needle has a cutting tip

18 Ethylene oxide:

- a Is commonly used for sterilization of most anaesthetic equipment
- b Is a non-toxic gas
- c Does not require special equipment when used for sterilization
- d Can be used for sterilization of plastic
- e Is less expensive than steam sterilization

19 A Hickman catheter:

- a Is made of polyvinyl chloride (PVC)
- b Has a subcutaneous Dacron cuff
- c Is available as a single- or multi-lumen catheter
- d Are used for haemodialysis
- e Should be changed every six weeks if required for long-term use

20 Concerning impedance:

- a It is the sum of forces that oppose the movement of electrons in a DC circuit
- b The unit for impedance is the coulomb
- c The term impedance covers resistors, capacitors, and inductors, and is dependent on the frequency of the current
- d Substances with high impedance are termed insulators
- e The change in impedance in the chest wall during a cardiac systole is the principle used in impedance plethysmography to measure cardiac output

21 Regarding Wright's respirometer:

- a It is a device that measures the tidal and minute volume
- b It has a rotating vane with a pointer attached to it
- c The vane does 100 revolutions for every litre of air passing through
- d It is usually positioned on the inspiratory limb of the breathing circuit
- e It is accurate to 5–10% of the flow within the range of 4–24 l/min

22 Regarding a capacitor:

- a Capacitance is a measure of the ability of a conductor or system to store an electric charge
- b It consists of two parallel insulating plates separated by a conductor
- c The unit of capacitance is the farad (F)
- d Defibrillators store the energy in a capacitor.
- e It will allow direct current to flow in preference to alternating current

23 Static electricity in the operating theatre:

- a Can cause sparks, fire, and explosions
- b Can be minimized by keeping the relative humidity at 30%
- c Can be prevented if the temperature is kept below 20°C
- d Is minimized if the floor is made of conductive material
- e Can lead to inaccuracies in gas flow measurement

24 Regarding bispectral index (BIS) monitoring of depth of anaesthesia:

- a A BIS monitor is a device to monitor the electrical activity and the level of sedation in the brain, and assess the risk of awareness
- b BIS reading is displayed on a 0–100 scale, the higher value indicating greater sedation
- c Hypothermia causes a lower BIS reading
- d Hypocapnia produces a low BIS reading
- e Is less sensitive to the analgesic than the hypnotic component of an anaesthetic

25 A catheter mount:

- a Links the airway device to the breathing system
- b Varies in length from 20 mm to 40 mm
- c Adds 25–60 ml to the dead space
- d Can allow suction of the trachea without disconnection from the breathing system
- e Has one end that fits a 22 mm connector

26 The Lack breathing system:

- a Is an example of a Mapleson D circuit
- b Is a coaxial circuit
- c Requires a fresh gas flow of 100 ml/kg/min
- d Is also available in a parallel tubing version instead of co-axial tubes
- e Is suitable for controlled ventilation

27 Supraglottic airway devices:

- a All use an air-filled cuff
- b May be used to drain gastric secretions
- c Should not be used in children less than 2 years old
- d Must be single use if used for tonsil surgery
- e Of the classic LMA™ variety are available up to size 7

28 Needles used for nerve blocks:

a Are made of steel
b Have short blunt bevels in order to minimize trauma to the nerve
c The optimum size is 18 G
d Vary in length from 2.5 cm to 15 cm
e Are coated with Teflon® over their entire length to insulate them

29 The severity of an electric shock is dependent on:

a The type of current, AC or DC
b The size of the current
c The duration of contact
d The frequency of the current
e The pathway the current takes through the body

30 The intra-aortic balloon pump:

a Involves threading a catheter via the vena cava into the left side of the heart
b Is inflated during systole
c Is contraindicated in severe cardiogenic shock
d Utilizes a 50 ml balloon filled with medical air
e Should not be used immediately following cardiac bypass

chapter 4

PHYSICS

ANSWERS

1 During invasive arterial pressure monitoring:

a **True** Soft cannulae become even softer when *in situ* due to the effect of body heat and may contribute to the poor reproduction of the waveform.

b **False** The catheter should not be longer than 2 m in length preferably.

c **False** A soft diaphragm would contribute to damping.

d **True** It is the difference between the systolic and diastolic pressures whereas the mean arterial pressure is diastolic plus one-third of the pulse pressure.

e **True** In order to be able to display the arterial waveform correctly the system should be capable of responding to a frequency range of 0.5–40 Hz as this is the frequency range of the arterial pressure wave.

Al-Shaikh B and Stacey S (2006) *Essentials of Anaesthetic Equipment*, 3rd edition. Edinburgh: Churchill Livingstone.

Davis P and Kenny G (2002) *Basic Physics and Measurement in Anaesthesia*, 5th edition. Boston, MA: Butterworth-Heinemann.

2 The pneumotachograph:

a **True** The pneumotachograph measures gas flow and can also be used to measure gas volume from this.

b **False** The Wright respirometer measures volume from unidirectional gas flow only. The pneumotachograph can measure flows both in inspiration and expiration.

c **True** The pneumotachograph has a gauze screen which acts as a resistance to gas flow. Gas flow causes a small pressure drop across the gauze, which is measured by a transducer. The pressure drop is linearly proportional to the flow rate of gas within a certain range.

d **True** The resistance is provided by the gauze screen or a bundle of parallel tubes; the flow through the gauze or screen is laminar.

e **True** As with most devices measuring respiratory flows, condensation of water vapour can increase the resistance and cause inaccuracies. This problem is overcome by heating the gauze or parallel tubes.

Al-Shaikh B and Stacey S (2006) *Essentials of Anaesthetic Equipment*, 3rd edition. Edinburgh: Churchill Livingstone.

3 Concerning ventilator alarms:

a **True** Measurement of peak inspiratory pressure or the expired volume is the principle used in these devices

b **False** The device measures changes in inspiratory pressure and hence it is connected to the inspiratory limb. A sudden decrease in pressure can indicate disconnection and an increase could mean obstruction.

c **True** The changes in the expired volume are designed to trigger the alarm.

d **False** They are connected to the expiratory limb of the circuit.

e **True** These alarms form part of essential monitoring required during artificial ventilation.

Al-Shaikh B and Stacey S (2006) *Essentials of Anaesthetic Equipment*, 3rd edition. Edinburgh: Churchill Livingstone.

Davis P and Kenny G (2002) *Basic Physics and Measurement in Anaesthesia*, 5th edition. Boston, MA: Butterworth-Heinemann.

4 Regarding peripheral nerve stimulators:

a **False** The two electrodes are placed over the nerve with the negative electrode distally and the positive electrode 2 cm proximally.

b **False** They deliver a steady, constant current.

c **True** It is known as the train-of-four ratio. As the muscle relaxant is administered, fade is noticed first followed by disappearance of the fourth twitch, then the third, second, and first. During recovery the first twitch appears first and then the rest follow sequentially.

d **False** 50–100 Hz is used for tetanic stimulation to detect any residual neuromuscular block. Higher frequencies can cause severe discomfort to the patient emerging from anaesthesia.

e **False** Two short bursts of 50 Hz are applied with a 750 ms interval. Double-burst stimulation allows a more accurate assessment of residual block than train-of-four.

Al-Shaikh B and Stacey S (2006) *Essentials of Anaesthetic Equipment*, 3rd edition. Edinburgh: Churchill Livingstone.

5 Tympanic membrane temperature:

a **True** The small probe with a disposable cover is inserted into the external auditory meatus. The detector receives infrared radiation from the tympanic membrane which is converted into an electrical signal. The response time is about three seconds.

b **True** It is a true reflection of core temperature. Recovery time from cardiopulmonary bypass can be predicted from the brain temperature as well as the temperature of the heart estimated from an oesophageal probe.

c **False** Both tympanic membrane and lower oesophageal temperature correlate equally well with the core temperature.

d **True** The temperature probe may use a series of thermocouples, known as a thermopile, or a thermistor consisting of a small bead of metal oxide.

e **False** The temperature in the bladder is more accurate if there is adequate urine flow. It is not affected by changes in the ambient temperature.

Al-Shaikh B and Stacey S (2006) *Essentials of Anaesthetic Equipment*, 3rd edition. Edinburgh: Churchill Livingstone.

6 Nerve stimulators used for nerve blocks:

a **False** The negative lead is connected to the needle and the positive lead is connected to the an area of clean, dry skin of the patient to complete the circuit.

b **False** The duration of the stimulus is short, 1–2 ms to produce a painless muscle contraction.

c **True** A 2 Hz frequency allows more frequent feedback.

d **False** Peripheral nerve stimulators used to monitor neuromuscular block are high-output devices and can damage nerves if used for locating nerves for nerve blocks.

e **True** With a higher current muscle twitches can be elicited even if the needle is not close to the nerve. However, persisting muscle twitches at 0.2 mA indicate that the needle is potentially within the nerve or nerve sheath and should be withdrawn before injection of local anaesthetic.

Al-Shaikh B and Stacey S (2006) *Essentials of Anaesthetic Equipment*, 3rd edition. Edinburgh: Churchill Livingstone.

7 Continuous positive airway pressure (CPAP):

a **True** When the patient is being ventilated artificially, the term would be positive end-expiratory pressure (PEEP).

b **False** A pressure greater than 15 cmH_2O would cause a greatly increased resistance to breathing and would have adverse effects on venous return and could also cause barotrauma.

c **True** The increased intrathoracic pressure can decrease venous return and thus cardiac output.

d **False** Although patients tolerate the nasal masks better, mouth breathing reduces the effects of CPAP, making them equally or potentially less efficient.

e **True** Breathing spontaneously with CPAP causes less barotrauma to the immature lungs and allows surfactant production to begin. Usually the newborn recovers in just over 72 hours if surfactant production continues at a normal rate. Supportive therapy in the form of artificial surfactant is also available.

Al-Shaikh B and Stacey S (2006) *Essentials of Anaesthetic Equipment*, 3rd edition. Edinburgh: Churchill Livingstone.

8 Flow through intravenous cannulae:

a **False** 22 G allows 31–33 ml/min.

b **False** 20 G allows 40–80 ml/min.

c **False** 18 G allows 75–120 ml/min.

d **False** 16 G allows 130–220 ml/min.

e **True** 14 G allows 250–360 ml/min.

These figures are obtained using distilled water at a pressure of 10 kPa, through 110 cm long tubing with an internal diameter of 4 mm.

Al-Shaikh B and Stacey S (2006) *Essentials of Anaesthetic Equipment*, 3rd edition. Edinburgh: Churchill Livingstone.

9 Concerning intravenous (IV) administration of fluids:

a **False** Most standard adult giving sets are 4 mm in internal diameter.
b **False** Blood giving sets have a filter with a 150 μm mesh size. These filters are only able to filter out large clumps of red cells and other debris.
c **False** 20 drops of clear fluid = 1 ml and 15 drops of blood = 1 ml in adult giving sets.
d **False** 60 drops of clear fluid = 1 ml in paediatric giving sets.
e **True** Burettes used for paediatric blood transfusion produce 15 drops per ml. This provides the same drop size as in adult blood giving sets.

Al-Shaikh B and Stacey S (2006) *Essentials of Anaesthetic Equipment*, 3rd edition. Edinburgh: Churchill Livingstone.

10 The pH electrode:

a **True** It measures the activity of hydrogen ions in a sample. pH can then be calculated from the equation: $pH = -\log [H^+]$.
b **True** It can also measure the pH of other fluids such as pleural fluid and cerebrospinal fluid (CSF).
c **False** The pH electrode has a calomel (mercury/mercury chloride) reference electrode and a glass silver/silver chloride measuring electrode, which is a bulb of pH-sensitive glass containing a buffer solution.
d **True** The reference electrode has a constant potential. When a sample is introduced, hydrogen ions within the sample create a pH gradient between the sample and the buffer solution. An electrical potential is created at the measuring electrode. The two electrodes are connected to complete a circuit and the electrical potential produced is proportional to the pH of the sample.
e **False** 1 unit of pH produces a linear output of 60 mV.

Al-Shaikh B and Stacey S (2006) *Essentials of Anaesthetic Equipment*, 3rd edition. Edinburgh: Churchill Livingstone.

11 Defibrillators:

a **False** DC energy is more effective than AC energy therefore uses lower energy, causing less damage to the heart. It also has less potential for provoking arrhythmia.
b **False** A capacitor stores the charge ready for discharge. When the circuit is completed by closing both switches, the stored charge from the capacitor is delivered to the patient. The inductor absorbs some of the charge and modifies the current waveform delivered to the patient so that delivery of current to the myocardium is more efficient.
c **True** The conventional pad position is over the sternum and the left mid-axillary line.
d **True** The impedance to the flow of current is 50–150 ohms so only a small proportion of the current reaches the myocardium.
e **False** The shock is synchronized with the R wave of the ECG to prevent the R-on-T phenomenon, which can precipitate ventricular fibrillation or ventricular tachycardia.

Al-Shaikh B and Stacey S (2006) *Essentials of Anaesthetic Equipment*, 3rd edition. Edinburgh: Churchill Livingstone.
Yentis S, Hirsh N, and Smith G (2003) *Anaesthesia and Intensive Care A to Z*, 3rd edition. London: Butterworth-Heinemann.

12 Maintenance measures for gas cylinders include:

a **True** This keeps the nozzle free from dust and other particles.
b **False** Any grease or lubricant increases the risk of explosion.
c **True** Storage in a cold place ensures that the gases within do not expand excessively and risk an explosion, especially in tropical climates.
d **True** One cylinder from a batch is picked randomly for testing. One test consists of filling the cylinder with water under pressure to check for leaks. Other tests include the 'tensile test' and flattening, impact or bend tests where strips are cut from the cylinder and subjected to stretching and a crushing weight applied, respectively. Guidelines suggest 1 in 100 cylinders are checked.
e **False** Nitrous oxide is in the liquid form inside the cylinder, and ample room should be available for it to expand. The suggested filling ratio is 0.67 for hot climates, but in the UK the filling ratio is 0.75, therefore one may exceed the filling ratio of 0.69 (see Table 3.2).

Al-Shaikh B and Stacey S (2006) *Essentials of Anaesthetic Equipment*, 3rd edition. Edinburgh: Churchill Livingstone.
Kevin K and Spoors C (2009) *Training in Anaesthesia*. New York: Oxford University Press.

13 With regard to lasers:

a **False** Laser stands for light amplification by the stimulated emission of radiation.
b **False** The carbon dioxide laser is used for fine cutting and precision surgery, e.g. ENT and neurosurgery. It is also used for general, gynaecological, and dermatological procedures. The argon or krypton laser is used for photocoagulation in ophthalmic surgery.
c **True** They have a flexible stainless steel body. Reflected beams are defocused to reduce accidental laser strikes to healthy tissues.
d **True** An air filled cuff may ignite if hit by a laser beam and hence the recommendation of using saline instead of air to inflate the cuff, or alternatively to use an uncuffed tube.
e **True** Special goggles should be worn by all the staff and the patient. Carbon dioxide laser energy will be absorbed by glasses, but the other lasers require the use of tinted goggles.

Al-Shaikh B and Stacey S (2006) *Essentials of Anaesthetic Equipment*, 3rd edition. Edinburgh: Churchill Livingstone.
Yentis S, Hirsh N, and Smith G (2003) *Anaesthesia and Intensive Care A to Z*, 3rd edition. London: Butterworth-Heinemann.

14 Regarding latex and latex allergy:

a **True** It is a milky liquid derived from the *Hevea brasiliensis* rubber tree and is used in the manufacture of a vast array of medical and non-medical material and equipment.
b **True** A food allergy history should therefore be elicited from all patients in addition to drug allergies in the preoperative assessment.
c **True** Diagnosis can be made clinically, by skin prick testing, skin patch testing, or by RAST. RAST stands for radioallergosorbent test and is a blood test that aims to detect the amount of IgE present that reacts specifically with suspected or known allergens.
d **True** Anaesthetic and other equipment should be examined for a symbol indicating it is latex free before use.
e **True** Since most of the antibiotic vials have rubber stoppers, they should be removed away from the patient before reconstituting the drug.

Al-Shaikh B and Stacey S (2006) *Essentials of Anaesthetic Equipment*, 3rd edition. Edinburgh: Churchill Livingstone.

15 Regarding epidural needles:

a **False** The needle most commonly used in adults is 16 G and 10 cm long.
b **False** The bevel is at 20° to the shaft.
c **True** Huber was the person who developed the needle which Tuohy popularized and is now more commonly known by the latter name.
d **False** A 15 cm version is available in the UK for use in obese patients.
e **True** A 19 G needle of 5 cm length is used in paediatric practice. It allows the passage of a 21 G epidural catheter.

Al-Shaikh B and Stacey S (2006) *Essentials of Anaesthetic Equipment*, 3rd edition. Edinburgh: Churchill Livingstone.

16 Epidural catheters:

a **False** They are 90 cm long, they are made of nylon or Teflon, and they are biologically inert.
b **False** The external diameter of the catheter is 1 mm and the internal diameter is 0.5 mm.
c **True** Some designs are radio-opaque.
d **True** This practice risks shearing off part of the catheter and leaving it within the epidural space. If the catheter needs to be removed at this stage, both the Tuohy needle and the catheter should be withdrawn as one unit.
e **True** The filter has a 0.22 μm mesh which prevents the injection of bacteria, viruses, and pieces of glass ampoule or other foreign material into the epidural space. The filter may need replacing if the epidural is in place for a prolonged period.

Al-Shaikh B and Stacey S (2006) *Essentials of Anaesthetic Equipment*, 3rd edition. Edinburgh: Churchill Livingstone.

17 Concerning spinal needles:

a **False** Most anaesthetists use a 25 G needle or smaller for spinal anaesthesia and only use the bigger needles for difficult cases.
b **False** The most commonly used needles are 10 cm long. They are also available in 5 cm or 15 cm lengths.
c **True** This prevents bending or kinking of the spinal needle which occurs with the 25 G or smaller needles. The 22 G more rigid needle used for difficult cases and can be inserted without the introducer.
d **True** The cutting point needles, e.g. Quincke and Yale, cut the dural fibres and are more likely to result in postdural puncture headache than the pencil point designs, which push the fibres apart atraumatically.
e **False** The Whitacre and Sprotte needles have a pencil point with a preterminal side-hole. They are less traumatic.

Al-Shaikh B and Stacey S (2006) *Essentials of Anaesthetic Equipment*, 3rd edition. Edinburgh: Churchill Livingstone.

18 Ethylene oxide:

a **True** Ethylene oxide is relatively cheap compared with other methods and it does not damage plastics and rubber, so despite its disadvantages it remains in common use.

b **False** It is extremely toxic so a long period, up to two weeks, of aeration is required before the sterilized equipment can be used.

c **False** It is an explosive gas and special equipment is required for its use.

d **True** Most equipment that can withstand temperatures of 50–60°C can be sterilized using ethylene oxide. It can be difficult to eradicate all traces of ethylene oxide from plastic and rubber equipment.

e **False** It is extremely expensive, but may be the only method available for sterilizing some equipment that would be damaged by other processes, e.g. dry heat or autoclaving. It is less expensive than gamma irradiation techniques.

Al-Shaikh B and Stacey S (2006) *Essentials of Anaesthetic Equipment*, 3rd edition. Edinburgh: Churchill Livingstone.

19 A Hickman catheter:

a **False** Is made of polyurethane or silicone.

b **True** The cuff sits under the skin and induces a fibroblastic reaction that holds the tunnelled catheter in place. This also acts as a barrier to skin organisms.

c **True** They are available as a single-, double-, or triple-lumen catheter, depending on the indication for use.

d **False** The catheters used for haemodialysis are large-bore catheters. Hickman catheters are used for chemotherapy, long-term parenteral medication or nutrition and in paediatrics for repeated blood sampling and anaesthesia in the treatment of some cancers, e.g. leukaemia.

e **False** With suitable attention to hygiene when in use, Hickman catheters can stay *in situ* for several months without the need for replacement.

Al-Shaikh B and Stacey S (2006) *Essentials of Anaesthetic Equipment*, 3rd edition. Edinburgh: Churchill Livingstone.

20 Concerning impedance:

a **False** Impedance is the sum of forces opposing the movement of alternating current in an electrical circuit.

b **False** The unit of impedance is the ohm.

c **True** All different electrical equipment in use has an impedance.

d **True** Hence they present higher resistance to the flow of electricity. Substances with low impedance are referred to as conductors.

e **True** As the blood flows down the aorta during systole there is a change in impedance in the chest wall, which is computed to give the flow and the cardiac output.

Al-Shaikh B and Stacey S (2006) *Essentials of Anaesthetic Equipment*, 3rd edition. Edinburgh: Churchill Livingstone.

21 Regarding Wright's respirometer:

a **True** It allows measurement of tidal volume if the flow of gases is directed one way only.

b **True** The vane is surrounded by slits so that it may rotate in a circular motion.

c **False** The vane makes 150 revolutions for every 1 litre.

d **False** It has to be on the expiratory limb since it measures the expired tidal and minute volume.

e **True** A minimum flow of 2 l/min is required for the device to function efficiently.

Al-Shaikh B and Stacey S (2006) *Essentials of Anaesthetic Equipment*, 3rd edition. Edinburgh: Churchill Livingstone.

22 Regarding a capacitor:

a **True** Capacitance is a measure of the conductor or system to store a charge.

b **False** A capacitor consists of two parallel conductors separated by an insulator.

c **True** The farad is the capacitance of an object for which the electrical potential increases by 1 V when 1 coulomb of charge is added to it. Since the farad is large the microfarad is used in clinical practice.

d **True** The defibrillator uses a potential difference of around 5000 V across the two plates of the capacitor to store electrical charge. When required, via a switch, the stored charge is released as a current pulse delivered through the patient's chest and therefore heart.

e **False** A capacitor will allow the flow of AC in preference to DC. It also preferentially allows high-frequency current to pass as there is less time for the current to decay.

Al-Shaikh B and Stacey S (2006) *Essentials of Anaesthetic Equipment*, 3rd edition. Edinburgh: Churchill Livingstone.

23 Static electricity in the operating theatre:

a **True** This was more relevant in the days when explosive inhalational agents such as diethyl ether and cyclopropane were in use.

b **False** A relative humidity of over 50% is recommended.

c **False** Maintaining the temperature greater than 20°C reduces the build-up of static electricity.

d **True** The earthed current should not be allowed to build up on the floor. Other apparatus, e.g. tables and trolleys have conducting wheels to allow static to be carried away.

e **True** If static is allowed to build up inside the flow meter of the anaesthetic machine, it can lead to the bobbin sticking to the sides of the flow meter tube. For this reason some designs incorporate a conductive strip to dissipate the charge.

Al-Shaikh B and Stacey S (2006) *Essentials of Anaesthetic Equipment*, 3rd edition. Edinburgh: Churchill Livingstone.

24 Regarding bispectral index (BIS) monitoring of depth of anaesthesia:

a **False** It monitors the muscular (electromyographic or EMG) and the cortical activity using a single flexible sensor that is stuck to the patient's forehead and temporal region. It gives an indication of the state of sedation of the patient.

b **False** The reading is displayed from 0 to 100, the lower numbers denoting greater sedation. A reading of 0 equates to total sedation and 100 signifies an awake patient. A reading of 40–60 is considered acceptable for general anaesthesia without awareness.

c **True** Changes in body temperature would affect the reading.

d **True** Hypocapnia low enough to cause a decrease in cerebral perfusion would affect the BIS reading.

e **True** In addition, hypnosis with ketamine cannot be measured with a BIS monitor since ketamine causes a dissociative anaesthesia and has excitatory effects on the electroencephalogram (EEG).

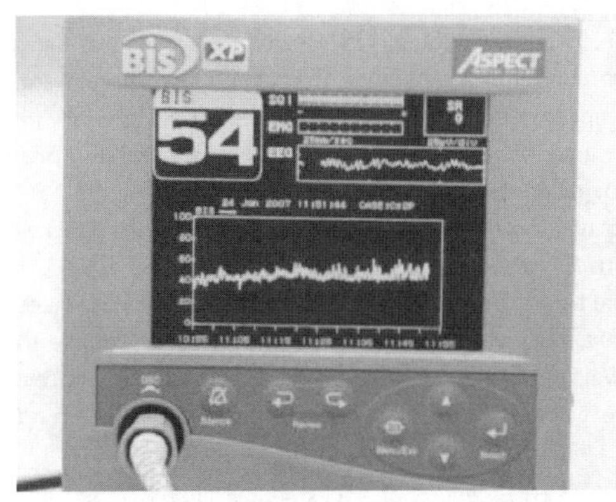

Figure 4.1 A bispectral index (BIS) monitor.

Al-Shaikh B and Stacey S (2006) *Essentials of Anaesthetic Equipment*, 3rd edition. Edinburgh: Churchill Livingstone.
Kevin K and Spoors C (2009) *Training in Anaesthesia*. New York: Oxford University Press.

25 A catheter mount:

a **True** It minimizes the transmission of accidental movements of the breathing system to the endotracheal tube or laryngeal mask.

b **False** The length varies from 45 mm to 170 mm.

c **True** This is of particular significance in paediatrics. Some mounts have a concertina design that allows the length to be reduced.

d **True** This is particularly useful during major surgery or care of patients in intensive care units. Bronchoscopy or suction can be performed without having to disconnect the ventilation tubing.

e **True** One end of the catheter mount has a 22 mm connector that attaches to the breathing system. The other end either fits a 15 mm standard tracheal tube connector or fits a 22 mm mask fitting.

Al-Shaikh B and Stacey S (2006) *Essentials of Anaesthetic Equipment*, 3rd edition. Edinburgh: Churchill Livingstone.

26 The Lack breathing system:

a **False** It is a Mapleson A, also known as a Magill breathing system.
b **True** The fresh gas flows through the outer tube and the expired gases flow through the inner tube.
c **False** A flow equal to the alveolar ventilation is required, which is 70 ml/kg/min. It is the most efficient circuit for spontaneous ventilation.
d **True** The fresh gas comes from one tube and expired gas is routed through the second tube.
e **False** Like its original version, the Magill breathing system it is not suitable for controlled ventilation.

Al-Shaikh B and Stacey S (2006) *Essentials of Anaesthetic Equipment*, 3rd edition. Edinburgh: Churchill Livingstone.

27 Supraglottic airway devices:

a **False** The i-gel is a supraglottic airway device that does not use an air-filled cuff. It is manufactured from a gel-like substance that moulds to the patient's larynx.
b **True** Several supraglottic airway devices, for example the LMA ProSeal™ and the i-gel, contain an integral channel for the passage of a gastric tube in order to decompress air in the stomach or drain its contents.
c **False** Supraglottic airway devices are available for use in children and neonates with sizes ranging from 1 (neonate up to 5 kg).
d **True** The Department of Health and the Royal College of Anaesthetists advise the use of disposable airway equipment for tonsillectomy to reduce the potential risk of transmission of variant Creutzfeldt–Jakob disease via prion proteins in lymphoid tissue.
e **False** The largest classic LMA™ available is a size 6, for use in adults weighing over 100 kg.

Al-Shaikh B and Stacey S (2006) *Essentials of Anaesthetic Equipment*, 3rd edition. Edinburgh: Churchill Livingstone.

28 Needles used for nerve blocks:

a **True** They are manufactured from steel, with a transparent hub to detect intravascular placement and a Luer lock attachment with injection tubing to allow an immobile needle injection technique.
b **True** Short bevelled needles also give a better tactile appreciation of the tissues as they are passed through various layers.
c **False** 20–22 G needles are the most widely used.
d **True** Where a nerve plexus is very superficial, e.g. brachial plexus from the interscalene approach, it is safer to use the shortest needle possible. The needle sizes commonly available are 2.5, 5, 10, and 15 cm.
e **False** The needles are coated in Teflon® except at their tip, which is left exposed to allow the current to flow and stimulate the nerve. This allows better localization of the nerve with a smaller current than if the current was spread over the entire length of the needle.

Al-Shaikh B and Stacey S (2006) *Essentials of Anaesthetic Equipment*, 3rd edition. Edinburgh: Churchill Livingstone.

29 The severity of an electric shock is dependent upon:

a **True** The direct current (DC) required to cause ventricular fibrillation is very much higher than with alternating current (AC).

b **True** A larger current causes more damage.

c **True** A shorter duration of contact causes less tissue damage.

d **True** The higher the frequency the less the damage; 50 Hz is the most lethal frequency, which is the standard AC frequency in the UK. The myocardium is most susceptible to arrhythmias at this frequency and muscle spasm prevents the victim letting go of the source.

e **True** Current passing through the chest may cause ventricular fibrillation and a current passing vertically through the body may cause loss of consciousness and spinal cord damage.

Al-Shaikh B and Stacey S (2006) *Essentials of Anaesthetic Equipment*, 3rd edition. Edinburgh: Churchill Livingstone.

30 The intra-aortic balloon pump:

a **False** A catheter is inserted percutaneously, usually via the femoral artery, into the descending aorta.

b **False** The balloon is inflated during early diastole. An increase in peak diastolic pressure occurs thus improving coronary perfusion pressure. Inflation is timed with the dicrotic notch of the arterial pressure waveform trace, coinciding with the period immediately following closure of the aortic valve.

c **False** Severe cardiogenic shock is one of the indications for the use of the intra-aortic balloon pump, where it reduces the myocardial oxygen demand and increases coronary artery perfusion. Other indications include imminent myocardial ischaemia, high-risk angiography, refractory unstable angina and arrhythmias associated with ischaemia.

d **False** The balloon is usually 40 ml or 34 ml in a small adult. It is filled with helium. If it was to rupture, 40 ml of air would present a significant air embolus.

e **False** Failure to wean from cardiopulmonary bypass, for example after coronary artery bypass surgery is one of the indications for the use of the intra-aortic balloon pump. Caution must be exercised if there is severe coagulopathy.

Al-Shaikh B and Stacey S (2006) *Essentials of Anaesthetic Equipment*, 3rd edition. Edinburgh: Churchill Livingstone.

chapter 4

PHYSIOLOGY

QUESTIONS

1 Concerning proteins:

- a All naturally occurring proteins are in the D-form
- b They catalyse chemical reactions
- c Albumin binds basic drugs in the blood
- d Are a key component of the immune system
- e Are involved in the transport of molecules and ions around the body

2 The sodium pump:

- a Exchanges intracellular sodium for extracellular potassium
- b Is important in maintaining constant cell volume
- c Is an example of an ion channel
- d Is inhibited in stored blood causing higher intracellular sodium in the red blood cells than potassium
- e Can be made to work efficiently by warming the cold blood back to 37°C

3 The resting membrane potential of a muscle fibre is:

- a The potential difference across the cell membrane during a muscular contraction
- b –90 mV
- c Dependent on the Gibbs–Donnan effect
- d +40 mV
- e Determined by the potassium equilibrium potential

4 In the central nervous system (CNS):

- a Grey matter consists of myelinated nerve axons
- b White matter consists of cell bodies of neurones
- c Oligodendrocytes form the myelin sheath in the peripheral nerves and Schwann cells form the myelin sheath in the central nerves
- d The axon is the main carrier of information to other neurones or muscles
- e After leaving the CNS the axons run in peripheral nerve trunks that provide structural support

5 A synapse:

- a Occurs when an axon reaches its target cell
- b Transmits information to the postsynaptic cell
- c Is a unidirectional system
- d Separates the presynaptic and postsynaptic membranes with a 5–10 nm synaptic cleft
- e The synaptic cleft stores numerous vesicles called synaptic vesicles

6 Neurotransmitters include:

a Acetylcholine
b 5-hydroxytryptamine (5HT)
c Gamma aminobutyric acid (GABA)
d Nitric oxide
e Enkephalins

7 The trigeminal nerve:

a Is a mixed nerve
b Arises in the lateral medulla
c Expands to form a ganglion
d Forms the efferent limb of the oculo-cardiac reflex
e Supplies the orbicularis oculi

8 Concerning pain:

a Nociceptive fibres are small diameter afferents that subserve pain sensation in a particular region
b Pinprick pain is conveyed by C fibres
c Pain sensation is carried in the dorsal columns to the sensory cortex
d Electrical stimulation of the peripheral nerves has been used to relieve pain
e Visceral pain is carried by lower thoracic and all the lumbosacral segments

9 Cardiac output is increased by:

a A rise in venous filling pressure
b A rise in body temperature
c Up to 700% during heavy exercise
d Eating
e High environmental temperature

10 The knee jerk:

a Is an example of stretch reflex
b Is a monosynaptic reflex
c Involves gamma motor neurons which are responsible for the contraction of quadriceps muscle when the patellar tendon is stretched with a sharp tap
d Is lost if the lower thoracic and upper lumbar segments are damaged
e Is absent in hypermagnesaemia

11 Regarding sickle cell disease:

a Haemoglobin levels are in the region of 6–9 g/dl in sickle cell disease
b In sickle cell disease the haemoglobin beta chains are normal but alpha chains are abnormal
c The Sickledex test is positive both in the disease and trait
d The haemoglobin level and the blood film are in the normal range in sickle cell trait
e HbS levels are less than 50% in sickle cell trait

12 Concerning haemoglobin:

- a Each gram takes up 1.64 ml of oxygen
- b Cyanosis is present if there is >2.5 g/100ml of deoxygenated haemoglobin
- c Each molecule of haemoglobin carries four molecules of oxygen
- d It is an important buffer in its reduced form
- e There is an iron molecule in the centre surrounded by four haem groups

13 Regarding the pituitary gland:

- a The posterior pituitary is known as the adenohypophysis
- b Hypophyseal portal vessels carry hormones from the hypothalamus, which controls the release of pituitary hormones
- c The anterior pituitary is in direct neural contact with the hypothalamus
- d Diabetes insipidus is caused by a lack of vasopressin
- e Thyrotropin is also known as thyroid-stimulating hormone (TSH)

14 Regarding the thirst mechanism in control of fluid intake:

- a It is mediated by osmoreceptors situated in the posterior pituitary
- b When serum osmolality increases by 4 osmol/kg thirst is stimulated
- c A decrease in circulating volume as seen after diarrhoea or haemorrhage stimulates thirst
- d The stretch receptors in the stomach limit fluid intake
- e Antidiuretic hormone (ADH) secretion controls the water intake

15 Features of primary hyperaldosteronism include:

- a An increase in serum sodium levels
- b Peripheral oedema
- c Hypocalcaemia
- d Muscle weakness
- e Hypoglycaemia

16 In the ABO blood groups:

- a Group A contains agglutinogen A and anti-B agglutinin
- b Group A is present in 60% of the UK population
- c Group B is present in 3% of the UK population
- d Group O has no agglutinogen but contains both anti-A and anti-B agglutinins
- e Administration of anti-D immunoglobulin (IgG) assists in the removal of anti-Rhesus antibodies from the plasma of a Rhesus-negative mother after delivery

17 The plasma of a normal adult:

- a Is 95% water
- b Has an osmolality of 270 mosm/kg
- c Contains most of the clotting factors
- d Accounts for 10% of body weight
- e Contains proteins in a concentration of 50–60 g/l

18 In the electrocardiogram (ECG):

a Electrical activity of the heart is measured
b Leads I, II, and III are known as unipolar limb leads
c Repolarization away from a lead results in a negative deflection
d Artefact may be produced by skeletal muscle activity
e Lead II records the excitation moving from the right upper portion of the heart to the tip of the left ventricle

19 Concerning skeletal muscle:

a Muscle fibres contain myofibrils, which are made of sarcomeres, the contractile units
b Contractile proteins in the sarcomeres are actin and myosin
c Sarcomeres are separated from each other by Z lines and consist of I and A bands
d The A band consists mainly of actin and the I bands contain myosin
e Troponin and tropomyosin contained in the muscles prevent the actin and myosin interacting continuously

20 Regarding distribution of blood in an adult at rest:

a Blood volume is approximately 5 litres
b 3–3.5 litres is contained in the capacitance vessels and large veins
c 600 ml is contained within the pulmonary circulation
d 10% is contained in the heart
e 20% is in the peripheral arteries

21 Coronary blood flow:

a Is maximal during ventricular diastole
b Varies according to the rise and fall in aortic pressure
c Is mediated by local metabolites
d Flow can increase by between 200% and 300% as a result of local hyperaemia caused by metabolic activity
e The PO_2 of the blood in the coronary sinus is about 2.7 kPa indicating high-normal oxygen extraction

22 Concerning muscle contraction:

a The basic element of motor control is the 'motor unit'
b Proprioceptors are mechanoreceptors situated within muscles and joints
c Cardiac muscle fibres cannot exhibit tetanic contraction
d Gamma motor neurones supply the muscle spindles
e Muscle spindles primarily measure the tension of a muscle while the tendon organs measure the length

23 Concerning the cerebral circulation:

- a It is approximately 15% of the cardiac output
- b It is increased by hypercarbia
- c It may cause syncope if the PCO_2 is reduced to around 3 kPa by voluntary hyperventilation
- d Nitric oxide released by the vascular endothelium increases cerebral blood flow
- e Cushing's reflex is a rise in blood pressure brought about in response to a rise in intracranial pressure (ICP)

24 Regarding cerebrospinal fluid (CSF):

- a Approximately 150 ml is formed daily
- b Around 20 ml is intrathecal
- c Reabsorption is proportional to CSF pressure
- d It has a higher pH than plasma
- e It contains no glucose

25 In the chemical control of respiration:

- a The carotid sinus and the aortic arch contain the peripheral chemoreceptors
- b The central chemoreceptors are situated in the pons
- c Central chemoreceptors respond to the pH of blood
- d The peripheral chemoreceptors only respond to the PaO_2
- e During anaesthesia the response to hypercapnia is increased

26 Growth hormone:

- a Is secreted by anterior pituitary gland
- b Release is controlled by growth hormone releasing hormone from the hypothalamus
- c Shows a diurnal variation, the levels being highest during the waking hours between early morning to midday
- d Is important for skeletal growth between 3 years of age to puberty
- e Deficiency may be accompanied by lack of pituitary hormones, notably TSH and gonadotrophins

27 Renal blood flow:

- a Is 25% of the cardiac output
- b To the renal cortex is twice the blood flow to the renal medulla
- c Is autoregulated at a mean arterial pressure of 180 mmHg
- d Can be maintained even if the nerve supply is severed
- e Is affected by local mediators such as prostaglandins and nitric oxide

28 Concerning urine production:

- a The proximal convoluted tubule reabsorbs all of the filtered glucose and amino acids
- b Water is actively reabsorbed in the proximal convoluted tubule
- c The loop of Henle creates an osmotic gradient in the renal medulla
- d The distal tubules reabsorb sodium and other ions and secrete hydrogen ions to acidify the urine when necessary
- e The collecting ducts reabsorb water under the influence of ADH, depending on the osmolality of the fluid reaching them

29 Concerning waveforms reflecting cardiac events:

a The 'a' wave in the neck corresponds to atrial systole
b The 'v' wave in the neck denotes ventricular systole
c The dicrotic notch of the arterial wave represents closure of the aortic valve
d The 'P' wave of the ECG occurs with atrial systole
e The 'U' wave in the ECG occurs with ventricular diastole

30 Interruption of the sympathetic supply to the eye causes:

a Dilation of the pupil
b Drooping of the eye lid
c Coldness of the side of face
d Lack of sweating on the affected side of face
e Anosmia

chapter
4

PHYSIOLOGY

ANSWERS

1 Concerning proteins:

a **False** All naturally occurring amino acids are in the laevo or L-form.

b **True** All catalytic reactions are mediated by enzymes that are proteins. Examples of important enzymes in respiratory physiology are carbonic anhydrase and cytochrome oxidase.

c **False** Albumin binds acidic drugs, e.g. thiopental (thiopentone), phenytoin, warfarin, and aspirin. Alpha 1 acid glycoprotein binds basic drugs, e.g. local anaesthetics, propranolol and quinidine. Globulins are also present in the blood and bind other drugs, e.g. tubocurarine.

d **True** Immunoglobulins are proteins that are important for fighting infection.

e **True** Protein binding is important in the transport of many substances, for example bilirubin, minerals, ions, hormones, and drugs.

Barrett K, Barman S, Boitano S, and Brooks HL (2009) *Ganong's Review of Medical Physiology*, 23rd edition. USA: McGraw-Hill.
Yentis S, Hirsh N, and Smith G (2003) *Anaesthesia and Intensive Care A to Z*, 3rd edition. London: Butterworth-Heinemann.

2 The sodium pump:

a **True** The sodium/potassium pump is present in every cell membrane and is responsible for the active transport of three sodium ions out of the cell and two potassium ions into the cells, establishing a negative membrane potential. This process is catalysed by an enzyme protein and uses the conversion of adenosine triphosphate (ATP) to adenosine diphosphate (ADP) to provide energy for the active process.

b **True** By maintaining the intracellular concentration of sodium the cell volume remains constant.

c **False** It is an example of a carrier protein that transports an ion or molecule against an electrochemical gradient, which requires energy from the hydrolysis of ATP. Hence it is an active transport system. Movement through ion channels always occurs down an electrochemical gradient and hence it is passive transport.

d **True** In stored blood potassium content is high, which is due to lysis of red cells and also due to inactivation of the sodium pump.

e **True** The use of blood warmers are especially important in massive transfusions for this reason to prevent hyperkalaemia.

Barrett K, Barman S, Boitano S, and Brooks HL (2009) *Ganong's Review of Medical Physiology*, 23rd edition. USA: McGraw-Hill.
Yentis S, Hirsh N, and Smith G (2003) *Anaesthesia and Intensive Care A to Z*, 3rd edition. London: Butterworth-Heinemann.

3 The resting membrane potential of a muscle fibre is:

- a **False** The resting membrane potential is the potential difference across the cell membrane when no stimulation is occurring.
- b **True** The resting membrane potential is dependent on the concentrations of charged ions, the permeability of the membrane to these ions, and the presence of ionic pumps. The resting membrane potential is –60 mV to –90 mV, being negative inside.
- c **True** The Gibbs–Donnan effect describes the differential separation of charged ions across a semipermeable membrane.
- d **False** This is the potential that is reached when an action potential is created. The potential rises to +40 mV before repolarization occurs.
- e **True** The resting membrane potential is determined by the potassium ion gradient because there are many more potassium ion channels open than sodium ion channels.

Barrett K, Barman S, Boitano S, and Brooks HL (2009) *Ganong's Review of Medical Physiology*, 23rd edition. USA: McGraw-Hill.
Cross M and Plunkett E (2008) *Physics, Pharmacology and Physiology for Anaesthetists*. Cambridge: Cambridge University Press.

4 In the central nervous system (CNS):

- a **False** The grey matter consists mainly of cell bodies of the neurones.
- b **False** It contains the myelinated axons and oligodendrocytes. Each cell body gives rise to only one axon but many branched dendrites, which receive information from many different cells. The axon ends in a single target cell.
- c **False** Oligodendrocytes form the myelin sheath in the central nerves and Schwann cells form the myelin sheath in the peripheral nerves.
- d **True** The axon is the main carrier of information and terminates in a specific receptor.
- e **True** This gives them the ability to traverse various parts of the body.

Barrett K, Barman S, Boitano S, and Brooks HL (2009) *Ganong's Review of Medical Physiology*, 23rd edition. USA: McGraw-Hill.

5 A synapse:

- a **True** A synapse occurs at the junction between a neurone (presynaptic cell) and another (postsynaptic) cell. The postsynaptic cell may be another neurone or a muscle or gland.
- b **True** There is electrical transmission of the action potential across the synapse.
- c **True** The action potentials travel in one direction only, controlled by the absolute refractory period of the neurone.
- d **False** The synaptic cleft is approximately 30–50 nm wide.
- e **False** The synaptic vesicles are stored in the presynaptic nerve terminal in a small swelling at the end of the axon also called the synaptic bouton or synaptic knob.

Barrett K, Barman S, Boitano S, and Brooks HL (2009) *Ganong's Review of Medical Physiology*, 23rd edition. USA: McGraw-Hill.
Yentis S, Hirsh N, and Smith G (2003) *Anaesthesia and Intensive Care A to Z*, 3rd edition. London: Butterworth-Heinemann.

6 Neurotransmitters include:

a **True** Acetylcholine is a neurotransmitter at autonomic ganglia, parasympathetic postganglionic nerve endings, sympathetic postganglionic nerve endings and sweat glands, and at the neuromuscular junction. Acetylcholine is involved in fast neurotransmission.

b **True** 5HT or serotonin is an amine neurotransmitter and is secreted in the peripheral and central nervous system as well as by smooth muscle and the gut. It is also found in platelets and mast cells. The amine neurotransmitters are involved in slow neurotransmission.

c **True** GABA is an amino acid neurotransmitter and is present in the brain and the spinal cord. The amino acids are involved in fast neurotransmission.

d **True** Nitric oxide acts in the brain as a neurotransmitter.

e **True** Enkephalins are polypeptide neurotransmitters and produce analgesia by reducing excitability.

Barrett K, Barman S, Boitano S, and Brooks HL (2009) *Ganong's Review of Medical Physiology*, 23rd edition. USA: McGraw-Hill.

Yentis S, Hirsh N, and Smith G (2003) *Anaesthesia and Intensive Care A to Z*, 3rd edition. London: Butterworth-Heinemann.

7 The trigeminal nerve:

a **True** The trigeminal nerve is primarily a sensory nerve of the face. It has more afferent fibres than efferent fibres.

b **False** It arises from the lateral aspect of the pons and has a small motor and a large sensory component.

c **True** Shortly after its origin it forms the trigeminal ganglion from which the three main branches—the ophthalmic, maxillary, and mandibular nerves—leave to innervate the face. These branches exit the skull via the superior orbital fissure, foramen rotundum, and foramen ovale, respectively.

d **False** The ophthalmic branch is the afferent limb and the vagus is the efferent. Traction on the ocular muscles or a sudden blow to the eyeball can lead to arrhythmias or asystole. The former is seen during squint surgery, particularly in the presence of hypoxia and hypercarbia. Asystole has been seen in boxers following a blow to the eye.

e **False** It is supplied by the facial nerve. The motor root of the trigeminal nerve supplies the muscles of mastication.

Barrett K, Barman S, Boitano S, and Brooks HL (2009) *Ganong's Review of Medical Physiology*, 23rd edition. USA: McGraw-Hill.

8 Concerning pain:

a **True** The perception of noxious stimuli is achieved by specialized nerve endings present within the skin and musculoskeletal system. These include C fibres, which respond to heat, mechanical, and chemical stimuli to produce pain, and A fibres, which respond to heat and mechanical stimuli, as well as cold.

b **False** Myelinated A delta fibres convey pinprick and sudden heat, and are responsible for rapid pain sensation and reflex withdrawal. Unmyelinated C fibres convey sensation of pressure, heat, and chemical tissue damage, and these fibres are also responsible for slow pain sensation and immobilization of the injured part.

c **False** First-order sensory neurones synapse within the dorsal horn, the second-order neurones cross over either within the dorsal horn or within a few spinal segments, and ascend within the anterolateral spinothalamic tract to the thalamus and periaqueductal grey matter. Third-order neurones then transmit pain from the thalamus to the somatosensory cortex.

d **True** This is the principle behind transcutaneous electrical nerve stimulation (TENS) and is based on the gate control theory of pain control. Stimulation of A beta fibres by high-frequency TENS and A delta fibres by low-frequency TENS inhibits pain transmission by C fibres.

e **False** Visceral pain is carried by the lower thoracic and upper two or three lumbar segments.

Barrett K, Barman S, Boitano S, and Brooks HL (2009) *Ganong's Review of Medical Physiology*, 23rd edition. USA: McGraw-Hill.

9 Cardiac output is increased by:

a **True** As preload increases, according to the Frank–Starling relationship, the filling of the ventricle causes an increase in the stroke volume and therefore in the cardiac output.

b **True** As body temperature rises, heart rate increases causing an increase in cardiac output.

c **True** During exercise cardiac output can increase by up to 700%; this is primarily achieved through an increase in heart rate as the stroke volume only increases to around twice resting value.

d **True** It is raised by up to 30% during eating.

e **True** The high environmental temperature raises body temperature and therefore cardiac output.

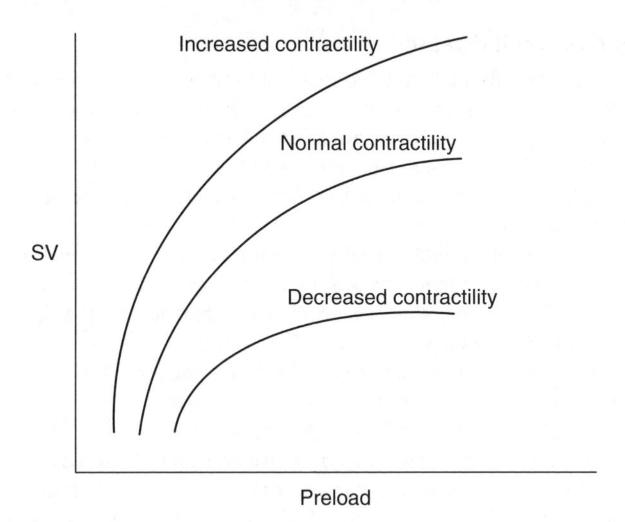

Figure 4.2 Frank–Starling curve.
Reproduced with kind permission from Kevin K and Spoors C (2009) *Training in Anaesthesia*. New York: Oxford University Press.

Barrett K, Barman S, Boitano S, and Brooks HL (2009) *Ganong's Review of Medical Physiology*, 23rd edition. USA: McGraw-Hill.
Waldman C, Soni N, and Rhodes A (2008) *Oxford Desk Reference: Critical Care*. Oxford: Oxford University Press.

10 The knee jerk:

- a **True** Stretching of the quadriceps tendon with the hammer blow increases the rate of firing of afferent group 1a fibres which causes the efferent alpha motor neurones at the spinal level to discharge and results in extension of the knee joint.
- b **True** The afferents from the muscle make monosynaptic contact with the alpha motor neurones to elicit a response.
- c **False** It is the alpha motor neurones which induce the contraction.
- d **False** The knee jerk is lost if the lower lumbar dorsal roots (through which afferents from quadriceps muscle pass) are damaged.
- e **True** Regular checking for the presence of the knee jerk reflex is helpful in assessing a patient treated with magnesium, in place of laboratory testing. At a plasma magnesium level exceeding 4mmol/l the knee jerk reflex is lost.

Barrett K, Barman S, Boitano S, and Brooks HL (2009) *Ganong's Review of Medical Physiology*, 23rd edition. USA: McGraw-Hill.
Yentis S, Hirsh N, and Smith G (2003) *Anaesthesia and Intensive Care A to Z*, 3rd edition. London: Butterworth-Heinemann.

11 Regarding sickle cell disease:

a **True** Anaemia is often present and levels of between 6 g/dl and 9 g/dl are common. This does not mean that transfusion is necessary, even when surgery is planned. Decisions regarding management should be discussed with a haematologist.

b **False** The alpha chains are normal but the beta chains are not. There is a valine residue instead of a glutamic acid residue in the sixth amino acid from the N-terminal of the haemoglobin beta chain.

c **True** This test involves adding a reagent to the blood and monitoring the turbidity. It is able to detect HbS but cannot make a distinction between sickle cell disease (HbSS) and sickle cell trait (HbAS), or other haemoglobin combinations. The differentiation can be made only by haemoglobin electrophoresis.

d **True** Normal or near normal haemoglobin levels and a positive Sickledex test gives a clinical diagnosis of sickle cell trait.

e **True** At a HbS level less than 50% the chances of sickling are minimal as the oxygen levels in arterial blood are unlikely to decrease enough to induce sickling (PaO_2 2.5–4 kPa). However, avoidance of hypoxia, dehydration, acidosis, and hypothermia should be the aim in the management of these patients as well.

Allman K and Wilson I (2006) *Oxford Handbook of Anaesthesia*, 2nd edition. New York: Oxford University Press.
Barrett K, Barman S, Boitano S, and Brooks HL (2009) *Ganong's Review of Medical Physiology*, 23rd edition. USA: McGraw-Hill.

12 Concerning haemoglobin:

a **False** Each gram of haemoglobin will bind 1.34 ml of oxygen at standard temperature and pressure.

b **False** Cyanosis will be evident if the deoxyhaemoglobin exceeds 5 g/100 ml.

c **True** Since there are four haem groups in a molecule of haemoglobin, it can combine with four molecules of oxygen.

d **True** Haemoglobin is an important buffer system in the body. It is most effective in its deoxygenated form when it can accept various waste products of tissue metabolism.

e **False** Haemoglobin contains four haem moieties. In the centre of each haem moiety there is one atom of ferrous (Fe^{2+}) iron that can combine with one molecule of oxygen.

Barrett K, Barman S, Boitano S, and Brooks HL (2009) *Ganong's Review of Medical Physiology*, 23rd edition. USA: McGraw-Hill.
Yentis S, Hirsh N, and Smith G (2003) *Anaesthesia and Intensive Care A to Z*, 3rd edition. London: Butterworth-Heinemann.

13 Regarding the pituitary gland:

a **False** The adenohypophysis is the anterior pituitary gland.

b **True** The hypothalamus releases pituitary-releasing hormones, which are conveyed through hypophyseal portal vessels.

c **False** Only the posterior pituitary has a direct neural connection with the hypothalamus.

d **True** Vasopressin is also called antidiuretic hormone (ADH). Diabetes insipidus is usually secondary to head injury or tumours affecting the pituitary gland.

e **True** Thyrotropin-releasing hormone from the pituitary causes release of TSH from the pituitary gland.

Barrett K, Barman S, Boitano S, and Brooks HL (2009) *Ganong's Review of Medical Physiology*, 23rd edition. USA: McGraw-Hill.

14 Regarding the thirst mechanism in control of fluid intake:

a **False** Osmoreceptors are situated in the anterior hypothalamus and lie outside the blood–brain barrier.
b **True** When the osmolality is increased osmoreceptors stimulate thirst and the behavioural response, which is to increase fluid intake, thus correcting the osmolality.
c **True** A decrease in extracellular and intracellular fluid occurs as the patient becomes more dehydrated, the osmolality will eventually increase if supplemental fluid is not given to correct the hypovolaemia. Stimulation of the osmoreceptors occurs and produces thirst.
d **True** The stretch receptors in the stomach limit the volume that can be ingested at any time.
e **True** Hypovolaemia is a potent cause of ADH release and also leads to activation of the thirst mechanism leading to an increase in fluid intake. ADH causes the collecting duct permeability to water to increase, leading to renal conservation of water. A small volume of dilute urine is produced. As the plasma volume increases and becomes more dilute, volume is conserved over plasma osmolality initially.

Barrett K, Barman S, Boitano S, and Brooks HL (2009) *Ganong's Review of Medical Physiology*, 23rd edition. USA: McGraw-Hill.

15 Features of primary hyperaldosteronism include:

a **True** Sodium and chloride levels rise. There is also hypokalaemia and metabolic alkalosis.
b **False** Despite sodium retention, peripheral oedema is not a feature.
c **False** Plasma calcium levels are unaffected.
d **True** Hypokalaemia may give rise to muscle weakness.
e **False** Blood glucose levels remain normal.

Barrett K, Barman S, Boitano S, and Brooks HL (2009) *Ganong's Review of Medical Physiology*, 23rd edition. USA: McGraw-Hill.
Yentis S, Hirsh N, and Smith G (2003) *Anaesthesia and Intensive Care A to Z*, 3rd edition. London: Butterworth-Heinemann.

16 In the ABO blood groups:

a **True** This means that a person with blood group A can accept blood of either type A or type O, but not AB or B.
b **False** Group A is present in 41% of the UK population; the most common is group O, which is present in 46% of the population.
c **False** Group B is seen in 10% of the population in the UK and AB in 3%.
d **True** This makes group O blood a valuable commodity as it is the 'universal donor'.
e **True** During delivery a Rhesus-negative mother may form antibodies in response to leakage of fetal cells into her circulation. Anti-Rhesus antibodies form and can complicate subsequent deliveries by causing haemolytic disease of the newborn if the mother gives birth to a Rhesus-positive baby. Administering anti-D immunoglobulin (IgG) after delivery will prevent the build up of these antibodies.

Barrett K, Barman S, Boitano S, and Brooks HL (2009) *Ganong's Review of Medical Physiology*, 23rd edition. USA: McGraw-Hill.

17 The plasma of a normal adult:

- a **True** Plasma is the non-cellular component of the blood and has a volume of 3500 ml in a 70 kg man.
- b **False** Normal osmolality is 280–305 mosm/kg.
- c **True** Most of the intrinsic pathway factors are present in the plasma.
- d **False** Blood volume accounts for 7–8% of body weight and plasma is about half of this or 4% of the body weight.
- e **False** Normal protein levels are 70–85 g/l. Albumin accounts for 45% and globulin, fibrinogen, and other proteins form the rest.

Allman K and Wilson I (2006) *Oxford Handbook of Anaesthesia*, 2nd edition. New York: Oxford University Press.

Barrett K, Barman S, Boitano S, and Brooks HL (2009) *Ganong's Review of Medical Physiology*, 23rd edition. USA: McGraw-Hill.

18 In the electrocardiogram (ECG):

- a **True** Cardiac electrical activity is recorded and displayed.
- b **False** They are known as the standard leads.
- c **False** Depolarization towards a lead, or repolarization away from a lead, results in a positive deflection. Depolarization away from a lead, or repolarization towards a lead, results in a negative deflection.
- d **True** Interference may be caused by skeletal muscle activity, e.g. shivering, or from diathermy or electrical equipment.
- e **True** Lead I records the activity along an axis between the right and left sides of the heart and lead III records the excitation spreading from the left atrium and the tip of the left ventricle.

Barrett K, Barman S, Boitano S, and Brooks HL (2009) *Ganong's Review of Medical Physiology*, 23rd edition. USA: McGraw-Hill.

19 Concerning skeletal muscle:

- a **True** Sarcomeres are the fundamental contractile units, the sarcomere shortens during muscle contraction.
- b **True** Each muscle fibre contains myofibrils, which contain actin and myosin filaments surrounded by sarcoplasmic reticulum and mitochondria.
- c **True** The sarcomere is between adjacent Z lines. The Z line is within the I band and the A band is between the Z lines. This is different from the cardiac muscle, where the cells are linked together by junctions called intercalated discs, which cross the muscle in irregular lines.
- d **False** The A bands consist mainly of myosin and I bands contain actin.
- e **True** These prevent a sustained contraction by the actin and myosin binding together continuously. When calcium ions are released from the sarcoplasmic reticulum, they bind with troponin on the actin filament, this in turn causes the tropomyosin complex to be displaced from myosin. The actin and myosin are then able to bind and the conformational change in myosin causes contraction of the muscle.

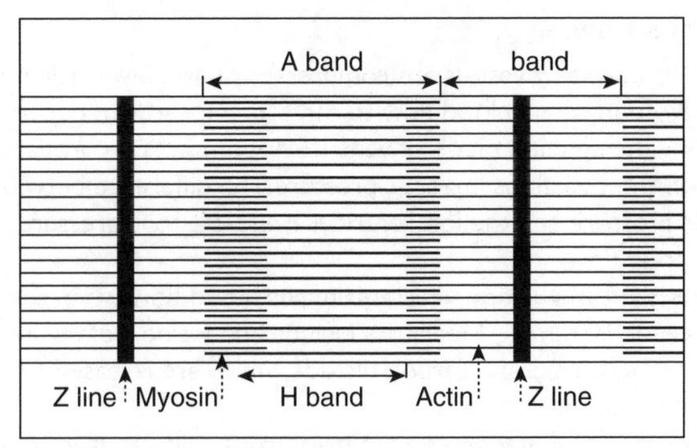

Figure 4.3 Simple diagram of skeletal muscle sarcomere, Z line, A and I band, actin, and myosin.
Reproduced with kind permission from Yentis S, Hirsh N, and Smith G (2003) *Anaesthesia and Intensive Care A to Z*, 3rd edition. London: Butterworth-Heineman.

Barrett K, Barman S, Boitano S, and Brooks HL (2009) *Ganong's Review of Medical Physiology*, 23rd edition. USA: McGraw-Hill.
Yentis S, Hirsh N, and Smith G (2003) *Anaesthesia and Intensive Care A to Z*, 3rd edition. London: Butterworth-Heinemann.

20 Regarding distribution of blood in an adult at rest:

a **True** In a neonate the blood volume is 90 ml/kg, this decreases to 80 ml/kg in a child and 70 ml/kg in an adult.

b **True** 60–70% of the blood distribution is within veins (capacitance vessels). This is why exsanguinating a limb prior to applying a tourniquet can present a sudden volume load to the patient that may not be tolerated, e.g. in cardiac failure.

c **True** Approximately 600 ml is held in the pulmonary vessels. When a Valsalva manoeuvre is performed, this blood is redistributed, causing a transient increase in blood pressure.

d **True** 10% of the blood volume is contained within the heart and 5% within the capillaries.

e **False** Peripheral arteries contain 10% of the total blood volume.

Barrett K, Barman S, Boitano S, and Brooks HL (2009) *Ganong's Review of Medical Physiology*, 23rd edition. USA: McGraw-Hill.

21 Coronary blood flow:

a **True** The left coronary vessels are compressed by the myocardium during ventricular systole therefore maximal blood flow to the subendocardium occurs during diastole.

b **True** During the ejection phase of ventricular contraction coronary blood flow is dependent on the variations in aortic pressure. The difference between the aortic end-diastolic pressure and the left ventricular end-diastolic pressure determines left ventricular blood flow.

c **True** There is autoregulation which maintains blood flow when the mean arterial pressure exceeds 60 mmHg. Mediators include adenosine, potassium, hydrogen ions, prostaglandins, lactic acid, and carbon dioxide, which are released from myocardial cells and cause vasodilation.

d **True** The release of metabolites from myocardial cells can lead to a threefold increase in blood flow during exercise.

e **True** Myocardial oxygen consumption is approximately 30 ml/min or 10 ml/100g/min. The oxygen extraction from the blood is 70% and any increase in demand for oxygen must therefore be met by increases in blood flow.

Barrett K, Barman S, Boitano S, and Brooks HL (2009) *Ganong's Review of Medical Physiology*, 23rd edition. USA: McGraw-Hill.
Yentis S, Hirsh N, and Smith G (2003) *Anaesthesia and Intensive Care A to Z*, 3rd edition. London: Butterworth-Heinemann.

22 Concerning muscle contraction:

a **True** The motor unit is one lower motor neurone and the muscle fibres innervated by the motor neurone. The fibres of the motor unit are all of the same type, e.g. fast or slow. The numbers of fibres per neurone varies depending on the site. For fine control, e.g. muscles of the face or hand there may only be a few muscle fibres supplied by each neurone, whereas for larger postural muscles one neurone may feed up to 1000 muscle fibres.

b **True** They provide the CNS with information regarding muscle length, position and tension.

c **True** As cardiac fibres have a prolonged refractory period they cannot undergo tetanic contraction.

d **True** In addition they receive Ia and group II afferent fibres.

e **False** Muscle spindles lie within the muscles and in parallel with skeletal muscle fibres and therefore can respond to muscle length and its rate of change. The Golgi tendon organs lie within the tendons and are in series with the contractile elements of the muscle. They are sensitive to the force generated within the muscle during contraction.

Barrett K, Barman S, Boitano S, and Brooks HL (2009) *Ganong's Review of Medical Physiology*, 23rd edition. USA: McGraw-Hill.
Yentis S, Hirsh N, and Smith G (2003) *Anaesthesia and Intensive Care A to Z*, 3rd edition. London: Butterworth-Heinemann.

23 Concerning the cerebral circulation:

a **True** Cerebral blood flow is 700 ml/min or 50 ml/100g/min, which is equal to 14% of the cardiac output.

b **True** The rising carbon dioxide leads to vasodilation and an increase in cerebral blood flow. When intracranial pressure (ICP) is raised to a critical level, deliberate hyperventilation of the intubated patient is sometimes used as a holding measure to reduce the ICP before definitive treatment, but this has a deleterious effect on cerebral perfusion.

c **True** Dizziness, visual disturbances, and loss of consciousness may occur due to the sudden decrease in cerebral blood flow caused by hypocapnia-mediated vasoconstriction of cerebral blood vessels.

d **True** Increased blood flow in response to hypoxia and hypercarbia is believed to be due to local release of nitric oxide from vessel walls.

e **True** As the brain is enclosed in the rigid skull a rise in ICP from any cause tends to lower cerebral blood flow and eventually forces the brain stem downwards through the foramen magnum. The resulting compression of the brainstem produces a marked rise in arterial blood pressure in a last desperate attempt to increase the cerebral perfusion pressure. This is known Cushing's reflex or response.

Barrett K, Barman S, Boitano S, and Brooks HL (2009) *Ganong's Review of Medical Physiology*, 23rd edition. USA: McGraw-Hill.

24 Cerebrospinal fluid (CSF):

a **False** The rate of production of CSF is 0.4 ml/min, over 500 ml/day. The total volume of CSF is about 150 ml. The majority (70%) is produced by the choroid plexuses within the cerebral ventricles. The remainder is produced by the endothelium of the cerebral capillaries.

b **False** Approximately a third to half of CSF is contained within the spinal theca, i.e. 50–100 ml.

c **True** CSF production is independent of CSF pressure, which is normally 112 mmH_2O in the lateral position. CSF reabsorption varies depending on the CSF pressure, rising pressure leads to an increase in reabsorption and when the pressure is less than 70 mmH_2O reabsorption ceases.

d **False** The CSF pH is same or lower than that of plasma. As the CSF contains very little protein, its buffering capacity is far less than that of plasma.

e **False** It contains between 2.7mmol/l and 4.8 mmol/l of glucose if the plasma glucose is normal. Glucose detection strips have been used to differentiate between saline and CSF to confirm suspected dural puncture during epidural insertion.

Aitkenhead A and Smith G (2008) *Textbook of Anaesthesia*, 5th edition. Edinburgh: Churchill Livingstone.

Barrett K, Barman S, Boitano S, and Brooks HL (2009) *Ganong's Review of Medical Physiology*, 23rd edition. USA: McGraw-Hill.

25 In the chemical control of respiration:

a **False** The carotid sinus and aortic arch contain the baroreceptors. The carotid and aortic bodies contain the peripheral chemoreceptors.

b **False** The central chemoreceptors are situated on the ventral surface of medulla.

c **True** The central chemoreceptors are stimulated by the hydrogen ion concentration within the CSF, which is related to increased carbon dioxide or metabolic acidosis. Oxygen has no effect on the central chemoreceptors.

d **False** The peripheral chemoreceptors are stimulated by a fall in PaO_2 and also by a rise in $PaCO_2$ and hydrogen ion concentration.

e **False** During anaesthesia, the respiratory response to hypercapnia and hypoxia is depressed. In a spontaneously ventilating patient, the carbon dioxide often rises with little change in respiratory rate, especially if opioids are administered.

Barrett K, Barman S, Boitano S, and Brooks HL (2009) *Ganong's Review of Medical Physiology*, 23rd edition. USA: McGraw-Hill.

26 Growth hormone:

a **True** This hormone is released in larger amounts than any other hormone from the pituitary gland.

b **True** The hypothalamus secretes growth hormone-releasing hormone (GHRH) which controls the release of growth hormone from the pituitary.

c **False** Growth hormone release is at its highest during the first few hours of sleep. Basal secretion during the day is low.

d **True** Inappropriate secretion of growth hormone in childhood is responsible for abnormal bone formation.

e **True** Lack of growth hormone can produce TSH and gonadotropin deficiency, and result in a mal-proportioned child who will fail to mature sexually. These effects can be reversed if replacement therapy is instituted promptly.

Barrett K, Barman S, Boitano S, and Brooks HL (2009) *Ganong's Review of Medical Physiology*, 23rd edition. USA: McGraw-Hill.

27 Renal blood flow:

a **True** Renal blood flow is 1200 ml/min or 22% of the cardiac output, despite constituting only 0.5% of the body weight. The kidneys are part of the vessel-rich group of organs.

b **False** Greater than 90% of the renal blood flow supplies the renal cortex, which receives 500 ml/min/100 g tissue whereas the outer medulla has a blood flow of 100 ml/min/100 g and the inner medulla receives 20 ml/min/100 g.

c **True** Between mean arterial pressures of 90 mmHg and 200 mmHg renal blood flow is independent of perfusion pressure, i.e. autoregulation occurs.

d **True** Autoregulation occurs even in denervated kidneys, for example renal transplants. The exact mechanism underlying autoregulation remains unclear.

e **True** These act as vasodilators and can increase blood flow when necessary. Non-steroidal anti-inflammatory drugs (NSAIDs) decrease levels of renal prostaglandins and where renal blood flow is compromised, this may lead to a large decrease in the glomerular filtration rate (GFR).

Barrett K, Barman S, Boitano S, and Brooks HL (2009) *Ganong's Review of Medical Physiology*, 23rd edition. USA: McGraw-Hill.
Pinnock C, Lin T, and Smith T (2002) *Fundamentals of Anaesthesia*, 2nd edition. New York: Cambridge University Press.

28 Concerning urine production:

a **True** In addition, most of the sodium, chloride and bicarbonate is reabsorbed in the proximal convoluted tubule.

b **False** The reabsorption of water occurs due to a chemical gradient in the tubule causing a small degree of hypotonicity. Another mechanism is differing permeabilities of bicarbonate and chloride, resulting in a net reabsorption of chloride and water, and some water is reabsorbed due to the presence of a hypertonic intermediate compartment, the lateral intercellular spaces.

c **True** This is accomplished by transporting sodium chloride from the tubular fluid to the interstitium without permitting the osmotic uptake of water.

d **True** Within the distal convoluted tubule, a further 5% of water is reabsorbed. Sodium ions are reabsorbed in exchange for either potassium or hydrogen ions. This process is under the control of the hormone aldosterone.

e **True** This absorption is water is active and essential in maintaining a constant osmolality of body fluids. ADH acts to increase the tubular permeability to water and therefore produces a concentrated urine.

Barrett K, Barman S, Boitano S, and Brooks HL (2009) *Ganong's Review of Medical Physiology*, 23rd edition. USA: McGraw-Hill.

Yentis S, Hirsh N, and Smith G (2003) *Anaesthesia and Intensive Care A to Z*, 3rd edition. London: Butterworth-Heinemann.

29 Concerning waveforms reflecting cardiac events:

a **True** The 'a' wave corresponds to atrial contraction.

b **False** The 'v' wave denotes the rise in pressure in the atria during filling before the opening of the tricuspid valve.

c **True** The transient upstroke in the descending arterial waveform represents a transient increase in pressure in the aorta and corresponds to closure of the aortic valve at the end of systole.

d **True** The P wave represents atrial depolarization and during this period atrial systole occurs.

e **True** The U wave is a small positive deflection following the T wave and is not usually seen except in sinus bradycardia, hypokalaemia, or after administration of quinidine and class 1a antiarrhythmics. Its significance is still not known.

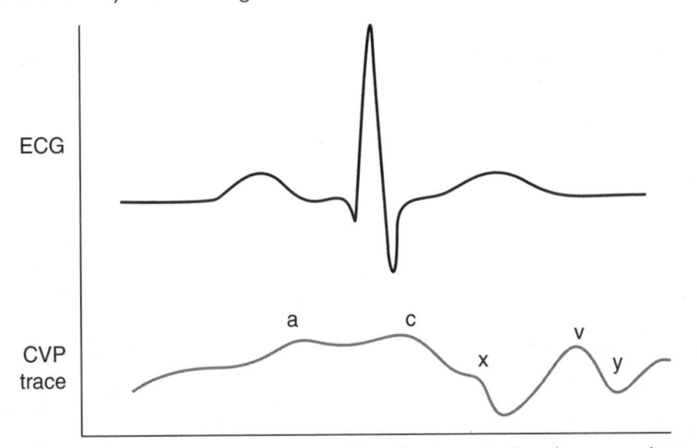

Figure 4.4 The central venous pressure trace with reference to the electrocardiogram.
Reproduced with kind permission from Kevin K and Spoors C (2009) *Training in Anaesthesia*. New York: Oxford University Press.

Barrett K, Barman S, Boitano S, and Brooks HL (2009) *Ganong's Review of Medical Physiology*, 23rd edition. USA: McGraw-Hill.

30 Interruption of the sympathetic supply to the eye causes:

a **False** Horner's syndrome occurs with pupillary constriction because of the unopposed action of the parasympathetic nerve supply to the pupil.
b **True** This is another feature of Horner's syndrome.
c **False** Vasodilation causes the area to be warm to touch.
d **True** Sweating is sympathetically mediated and does not occur.
e **False** Nasal congestion may be present on the affected side but this should not affect the sense of smell.

Barrett K, Barman S, Boitano S, and Brooks HL (2009) *Ganong's Review of Medical Physiology*, 23rd edition. USA: McGraw-Hill.

INDEX

MCQs FOR THE PRIMARY FRCA

Key: ■ denotes question, ■ denotes answer